DIET

A COMPLETE GUIDE TO
NUTRITION AND WEIGHT CONTROL

DANCING · AT · YOUR · PEAK

DIET

A COMPLETE GUIDE TO NUTRITION AND WEIGHT CONTROL

Robin D. Chmelar, M.S.
Sally S. Fitt, Ed.D.

Dance Books
9 Cecil Court
London WC2N 4EZ

Dance Books
9 Cecil Court
London WC2N 4EZ

Book Design by Susan Bishop
Cover Design by Main Street Design
Editorial Supervisor: Roxanne Barrett
Typesetting by Peirce Graphic Services

For Elizabeth R. Hayes
whose love of dance has inspired so many

Scientia est potentia
Knowledge is power

Contents

Tables

Figures

About the Authors

Robin Chmelar has divided her career among dance, writing, and health care. In the late '70s and early '80s, she was a member of Repertory Dance Theatre in Salt Lake City, where she also received her M.S. in Sports Medicine/Exercise Physiology and her B.F.A. in Modern Dance from the University of Utah. In addition, as an Associate Instructor for the University, she founded and developed a Dance Science course, from which much of the material for this book was derived. She is currently Research Specialist for Cybex, Division of Lumex, Inc. in New York, as well as an associate editor for *Kinesiology and Medicine for Dance.* Her research on dancers has appeared in *Medical Problems of Performing Artists, The Physician and Sportsmedicine, Journal of Orthopaedic and Sports Physical Therapy,* and *Dance Research Journal.* She has also written dance/health-related articles for *Dance Teacher Now, Network,* and *Center for Safety in the Arts,* and has been the recipient of a National Endowment for the Arts Choreographer's Fellowship.

Sally Sevey Fitt is a Professor of Modern Dance at the University of Utah in Salt Lake City, where she has taught since 1976. Her areas of specialization include dance kinesiology, movement behavior, and conditioning for dancers, and her recent book, *Dance Kinesiology,* has been called "a major contribution to both dance and exercise-science literature." She has received two Faculty Research Grants as well as the David P. Gardner Faculty Fellowship Award from the University of Utah. She received her doctorate from the University of California at Los Angeles, where she was also the recipient of the Chancellor's Fellowship. Her articles have appeared in such professional jorunals as *CAPHER Journal, AAHPERD Research Symposium,* and *Dance Research Journal.* Dr. Fitt has also collaborated with Robin Chmelar on studies of the physiologic characteristics of different styles and levels of dancers, the results of which have appeared in several journals.

Weight Control: A Dance Science Approach

For years, a talented young dancer struggled with her weight. There were always those extra five or ten pounds that kept her from making the leap from notable student to dynamic professional. She carefully followed diet after diet including those recommended by fellow dancers, teachers, and popular diet books, with typical up and down results. Ultimately it seemed that for every pound she lost, she would eventually regain two. In despair, she decided to give up dance and study sports science. However, an interesting turn of events took place through her studies.

Many of her sports science courses focused on the physiology of different types of exercise as well as diet and nutrition. Through her newly found knowledge, she began participating in different types of activities and drastically changed her eating habits. The result was a substantial weight loss and a significant change in her body proportions. She returned to dance, significantly leaner and stronger, and was soon hired by a major company.

What does this true story have to do with dance science? Mainly, it is that dance science and sports science focus on similar methods to achieve different goals. Whereas sports science takes the study of physiology, nutrition, kinesiology, motor learning, and psychology and applies them to the demands of sports, dance science takes these same components and applies them to the unique needs of dancers.

Dance science may be broadly defined as the systematic investigation of how the body responds to the musculoskeletal, physiological, and psychological effects of dance; that is, a scientific support mechanism for the *art* of dance. "Science" comes from the Latin word for "knowledge," and the purpose of dance science is to *support* the art of dance by offering greater knowledge. Dance science is intended to aid dancers in maintaining and improving the function of their instrument: their own bodies. A musician can have a piano maintained by a tuner but a dancer is the only person who can care for his or her body. Certainly, an intuitive feeling for the workings of the body is indispensable for the dancer; however, in certain cases this can lead toward unwise treatment unless it is balanced with a basic understanding of body facts and figures.

Communication regarding health and nutrition in dance is much like the game "Telephone." Because information is communicated primarily through word-of-mouth, much of it gets distorted, and when it comes to areas such as diet and nutrition, this distortion can cause a great deal of trouble.

There are many circles of nutritional beliefs, ranging from those who look at food intake in terms of maintenance of basic health to those who feel certain dietary measures can cure injuries or disease. One of our greatest challenges in writing this book was how to acknowledge the many diverse and contradictory nutritional theories, yet still provide meaningful information to the dancer. Often, what is of great interest to dietary experts is of no interest to dancers and vice versa. As a result, dancers tend to put their faith in fringe elements and advice from peers. However, our goal in this book is to synthesize scientific knowledge with real-life demands so that the information is useful on a truly practical basis. We feel dietitian Marilyn Peterson, who is the nutritional consultant for several dance companies, put it best with, "Although a strictly scientific approach may not always work [in dietary counseling of dancers], I have found that understanding them as individuals and gaining their confidence are often effective."

Most of the material in this book is based on the scientifically established work of nutritionists, exercise physiologists, and physicians; primarily research studies done on professional, university, and adolescent dancers. However, we have also tried to address certain areas that we have found to be of concern to dancers even though they might not fit into the traditional views of the above specialties. Some nutritionists may feel we have gone too far in our recommendations, while some dancers may feel we have not gone far enough, but such is the nature of the beast.

The nutritional information in this book will cover both general background information as well as how-to advice, but keep in mind that this advice will necessarily be general. We have also simplified a great deal of the material on physiology in order to get across those concepts of concern to the dancer without getting too bogged down in all the scientific "whys and wherefores." We realize that the metabolic and physiologic explanations don't give the whole story, but we have limited some of the information in order to keep it accessible to a wide range of dance readers.

We have also tried to use scientific journals as a major resource. While most journal articles concentrate on technical data, research on dancers' diets can certainly be translated into usable information for the dancer. With the help of such information, dancers should be able to make sound, well-informed decisions concerning their diet, which is exactly what we hope to promote. As the dancer mentioned earlier discovered, learning a few basics concerning diet and physiology can go a long way in getting the results desired for dance, as well as in improving overall health and fitness.

In addition, because of the demands for thinness in dance, dancers (especially females) usually need to strike a deal with food. Many female dancers have to restrict their caloric intake in order to be thin enough to perform, but if they don't eat enough or don't eat the right kinds of foods, their ability to perform suffers from fatigue and weakness. So, many dancers constantly vacillate between dieting to be thin and eating enough to maintain their energy, often with frustrating and unsatisfactory results.

In order to dance "at your peak," an appropriate balance between nutrition and weight control must be achieved, and the information in this book is intended to help you do just that. It is hoped that if dancers can gain greater knowledge about diet, physiology, and exercise they will have a greater understanding of how these components affect their dancing. And if you have greater understanding, ultimately you have greater control over your own health and performance.

Chapter I

Dieting, Weight Loss, and Dancers

The Dancer/Diet Phenomenon

"Dancers?" the exercise physiology researcher pondered when asked to compare them to athletes. "They're boring. All they ever talk about is food and how much they weigh." Such is the appearance of the dancer to many in the nondance world: obsessive, one-dimensional "thinaholics." Most dancers have a thorough repertory of dieting horror stories concerning either themselves or fellow dancers, and are all too familiar with dressing room talk such as, "All I had today was a grapefruit, some cheese, and a diet soda."

However, considering the kind of pressure exerted on the average female ballet dancer, it is no wonder thinness becomes an obsession. Since the unrivaled influence of Balanchine, the long-legged, wispy-thin look continues to be the aesthetic standard demanded by American ballet companies and schools. As for the modern or show dancer, although the demands for thinness may not be so severe, weight standards are nevertheless very low.

So what else is new? Dancers have known for years that theirs is an extreme lot in life when it comes to their bodies. Dancers *must* be exceedingly slender; you either cut it or you don't. So, the interest in diets, weight-loss schemes, and sauna pants continues unabated. One phenomenon in particular continues in full force: no matter how many books are published, no matter how much up-to-date research is reported by popular magazines, and no matter how many times one fad or another has ended in disaster, misinformation and just plain mythology concerning weight loss *abounds* in the dance world.

Although there is no shortage of diet books, they are not geared specifically for dancers, who need guidelines based on their unique needs and problems. By design, most of the research on which these books are based has been concerned with *over*weight (or, more correctly, overfat) people trying to achieve a *normal* body composition. When considering someone so obese that health is endangered, few traditional investigators can muster up much sympathy for the dancer with a normal body weight who must get even thinner. Not until recently have nutritionists and physiologists begun to seriously study the ultralean body compositions of elite dancers, gymnasts, and runners, and thus been able to provide some practical advice on how to deal with their body composition problems.

General diet and nutritional research does, however, increase our awareness of the underlying reasons for our thinness obsessions. Bennett and Gurin, authors of *The Dieter's Dilemma* (1982), state it most concisely with: "The central tenet of diet mythology is that thin people are *better* than fat ones—more beautiful, healthier, stronger of will." Any dancer who has ever been on the wrong side of the scale can certainly identify with the notion that it's not just the extra weight that is bad, but that somehow, as a person, you are a failure. Another basic assumption is that any responsible person can consciously control his or her desire to eat; therefore, anyone with a little willpower can eat less until the desired weight is achieved. If there is one thing the weight-loss research has shown, it is that eating behavior is not just a matter of conscious will nor some simple byproduct of Freudian neurosis, but rather a complex interaction of genetic, biochemical, hormonal, and psychosocial influences.

Common Myths (and Realities) About Weight Control

As part of our course in dance science at the University of Utah, the students (all of whom were dancers) were given a true/false test dealing with a number of weight-loss issues (an idea stolen, with his consent, from exercise physiologist Dr. Robert O. Ruhling). The test, of course, was rigged. Although many statements appeared true on first glance, all were actually false. What follows are some of these myths and their explanations:

1. If you would just maintain a reduced intake of calories, you'll lose weight easily and effectively until your desired weight is achieved.

Most of the students said they thought this wasn't true according to their personal experience; but everyone else always seemed to tell them otherwise (particularly instructors in goading them to lose weight). The fact is the body naturally tends to resist weight change and is especially adaptable to reduced-calorie situations. This probably goes back to our genetic origins when 7-11's were not so plentiful. In general, if you consistently reduce your caloric intake your body will try to adapt to that lowered amount. The body will slow down its metabolic rate, conserve energy, and try to maintain its mass on lesser and lesser amounts of food. There is a limit, of course, and people can and do starve themselves to death. However, the simple "calories-in-equals-calories-out" notion doesn't quite hold true. For the vast majority of us, the body is very adaptable to reduced food consumption.

The body usually does not adapt so elegantly to overconsumption of calories; that is, the body more easily gains weight than loses it (as if you didn't already know that). Genetic differences account for much of the variation in body fuel efficiency in that some individuals are naturally very "wasteful" and others are very "conservative" when it comes to food energy. The wasteful folks burn excessive calories just sitting around, the proverbial Jack Sprats of the world. These people have, among other things, an abundance of what are known in biochemistry as "futile cycles," which are literally the continuous production of energy even after the need for the energy has passed. Others have a paucity of these futile cycles and store fat like a can of Crisco. Although genetics may be a strong factor in all of this, diet and exercise can also significantly affect how "fast" or slow" your metabolism runs.

2. Exercise just makes you hungry and besides, you have to burn up 3,500 extra calories while you're exercising just to lose one pound.

First, the term "exercise" should hereby be banned in reference to general physical activity. Considering that exercise can mean anything from a walk around the block to a five-mile run, it is futile to lump all exercise into one category. Exercise can be classified by two basic criteria: intensity (how hard you work) and duration (how long you work). In general, high-intensity, short-duration activities (such as sprinting) are supplied by molecularly stored energy and glycogen (or sugar) stores in the muscle. Low-intensity, long-duration exercise (such as long-distance jogging or walking) relies primarily on the body's fat stores for fuel.

Now, about that 3,500 calories to burn off a pound of fat—while it is true that the average pound of fat is worth about 3,500 calories and it is true that running a marathon only burns up about 2,700 calories, just why do you think most of these elite distance runners are so skinny? Hint: the key phrase in the statement is "while you're exercising." One factor seems to be that endurance exercise helps speed up those futile cycles referred to earlier. Following endurance exercise, the body's metabolic rate will remain elevated for up to eight hours. So, extra calories are burned not only during the exercise session, but also while you're watching David Letterman, some six to eight hours later. In addition, exercise tends to maintain or increase the body's lean mass (muscle). While a pound of fat will do nothing to contribute to the body's metabolic rate (except in extra mass to lug around), a pound of muscle will increase the body's capacity to expend energy.

3. It's important to perform exercises like sit-ups and leg-lifts to help lose the fat around your stomach and thighs.

"Spot-reducing" exercises have never "melted" fat in specific areas and never will. "Spot" exercises do virtually nothing to burn fat in general. Although well-designed conditioning exercises are very important for dancers, even 100 of the most grueling abdominal curls a day will not make your stomach "flatter" unless accompanied by a loss of body fat.

There are primarily two locations for body fat, one surrounding the visceral organs and one underneath the skin (a small amount of fat also sheaths nerve tissue and exists in bone marrow, but that's not what all the *Cosmopolitan* articles are about). When one cuts into the gluteal area of a cadaver (particularly a fat one), one is met with mounds of greasy, yellow globs that closely resemble chicken fat. In anatomy lab, we used to slice off big hunks of the stuff before we ever got to the hip muscles. This graphic description is not intended to make you sick, but to emphasize the point that about 50 percent of the body's fat stores lie right on top of the muscles and even 10,000 leg lifts will not melt a specific pocket away. Exercise will tone the muscle underneath, but one would be wise to consider how much of that new muscle tone will show underneath several inches of yellow gunk. Endurance exercise combined with dietary modifications is the most efficient means of reducing fat anywhere on the body. Either that or a few thousand dollars worth of liposuction.

4. When you go on a starvation or very low calorie diet, first the body burns up its extra fat and then you start losing muscle.

Actually, the opposite is true. The body must have a constant level of glucose in the blood (i.e., blood sugar) to survive. Red blood cells can only live on sugar; no sugar, no red blood cells—no red blood cells, no you. The brain is also a big sugar eater; in fact, at rest, the brain consumes about 66 percent of the total circulating glucose supply (compared with only 40 percent of the oxygen). Generally, the brain requires about 100–145 grams of glucose a day which is equivalent to about 400–600 calories.

When sugar (or carbohydrate) intake is not enough to maintain a certain blood glucose level, the body must turn to its own muscle tissue (both visceral and skeletal) to supply the needed glucose. Fat molecules (except for a small portion of the molecule) cannot be converted to glucose molecules. So, in a starvation or low-calorie situation, the body must first break down its own protein stores to get the needed glucose. Skeletal muscle is the first to go, followed by the liver. Eventually the body adapts to the use of a byproduct of fat breakdown called ketones for fuel. As time goes on without food, fat breakdown increases and muscle breakdown decreases.

Now, all this may sound like a dandy way to lose weight. Starve yourself for three weeks, lose the fat and then build the muscle back up. Unfortunately, life is not that simple.

5. Going on a short-term high-protein, low-carbohydrate diet is the best way to lose fat.

It's a good way to lose water and muscle, but a lousy way to lose fat. The body reacts to a low-carbohydrate diet much the same way it reacts to starvation because ingested protein and fat cannot be used for body fuel like carbohydrates. In reality, approximately 75 percent of the weight lost during the first week on such a diet is water, with the rest coming mostly from muscle stores. This is due to the fact that when insufficient carbohydrates are ingested, the body must use its stores of glycogen for fuel, which are primarily in the muscles and liver. Because water is needed to store glycogen, when glycogen goes so does a great deal of water. In fact, muscle itself is about 72 percent water.

The *coup de grâce* occurs when one decides after a week or two of this diet to start eating carbohydrates again, even if total intake is still low in calories. The body first reacts by rebuilding its glycogen stores, which will restore the original pounds of water, and then some, in no time. Then the body starts rebuilding its depleted fat stores. The body has become much more energy efficient by this time so even a normal intake of food supplies excess calories, which are then stored as fat. People often berate themselves for regaining lost weight (and usually more) after one of these low-carbohydrate diets, thinking that they just can't control themselves. In reality, it is sort of biologic manifest destiny that the weight be regained. The body has *long* been skilled in survival and adaptation, much longer than we have tried to look good on stage in a yellow leotard.

6. Because dancers exercise so much, there's no excuse for being overweight. Overweight dancers just eat too much.

Dance is very physically and mentally exhausting, but the fact is it just doesn't burn very many calories. An average one-hour dance technique class utilizes about 200 kcal (calories) per hour for women and about 300 kcal per hour for men (Cohen et al., 1982c). You'd burn more calories with brisk walking the same amount of time. Our students would often respond to this by saying, "Are you *sure* that's all the calories a dance class burns?" We realize it sounds low, but here's part of the reason: dance is classified as a short-duration, high-intensity exercise; that is, dancers work very hard for short periods of time (one to three minutes) and then either rest or work at a very low intensity for a while before they do another short burst of high-intensity work. This type of activity depends primarily on muscle stores of glycogen for fuel, and simply does not burn very many calories. Fat cannot be used as fuel for high-intensity activity because, among other reasons, it cannot be broken down fast enough (see Chapter 2).

Although some dancers do chronically overeat or engage in

binge eating, most generally have a lower than normal caloric intake. Unfortunately, all this starvation dieting results in a great many undernourished, still overweight, frustrated dancers who impose a lot of unwarranted guilt on themselves.

7. Dancers who are thin enough to dance in a major company often have an eating disorder such as bulimia or anorexia nervosa.

"Ah-ha!" our students would exclaim. "Now this one *must* be true." Actually, recent research (Hamilton et al., 1986) has shown that eating disorders are more prevalent among relatively heavy dancers. That is, compared to other dancers, those who are heavier tend more towards disorders such as bulimia and anorexia nervosa than those who are thin. Bulimia is a syndrome characterized by ingesting large quantities of food followed by self-induced vomiting and/or laxative abuse. Anorexia nervosa is a psychiatric/physiologic disorder involving self-starvation, and dancers who suffer from it often end up heavier than when they started once they recover. Research shows that eating-disordered behavior *does not* lead to the thinner, leaner physique the dancer desires.

8. A pound of muscle weighs more than a pound of fat.

Trick statement. A *pound* of one thing cannot *weigh* more than a *pound* of another thing—think about it. Muscle has a greater density than fat; that is, one pound of muscle takes up less space than one pound of fat. The average pound of muscle occupies about 25 cubic inches of body area whereas a pound of fat occupies about 31 cubic inches. So, even if you lost five pounds of fat and replaced it with five pounds of muscle, you would weigh the same but be approximately 30 cubic inches smaller (see Chapter 3.)

It should be clear by now that losing weight and losing fat are not necessarily synonymous. Body weight is made up of a certain portion of bone, muscle, fat, water, and ash (inorganic minerals). The amount of weight we carry as fat is commonly referred to as percent body fat. No one can truly have zero percent body fat since a certain amount is essential for life. Men have less body fat than women, and active people have less than those who are sedentary. The average woman age 17–30 has a percent body fat level between 22 and 28 percent, while the average man of that age group has 12–16 percent body fat (Katch & McArdle, 1983, p. 129). In contrast, studies show that professional female dancers average 11–17 percent body fat, and male dancers average 5–11 percent body fat (Calabrese et al., 1983; Chmelar et al., 1988a; Cohen et al., 1985; Kirkendall & Calabrese, 1983; Micheli et al., 1984; Ryan & Stephens, 1989; White, 1982). (Most studies have been conducted on professional ballet dancers.) This does not mean that dancers' percent fat levels are unhealthy; it's just that the demands of professional dance require a very lean body composition.

Percent fat in university dancers is more difficult to assess because of the broad range of goals and demands in various programs. Preprofessional university dancers tend to have percent fat levels of 14–17 percent (Chmelar et al., 1988a), whereas general university dancers tend to be in the range of 18–23 percent (Dolgener et al., 1980; Haviland, 1978; Novak et al., 1978).

On a weight-loss program, one will usually lose some fat and some muscle as well, but the intent is to tip the scales in the direction of fat loss. Recent research has shown that a combination of endurance exercise and dietary modifications is superior to either exercise or diet alone in reducing body fat and total weight, as well as in maintaining those results.

9. In a well-balanced diet, ⅓ of the total caloric intake should come from protein, ⅓ from carbohydrates, and ⅓ from fat.

Nutritionists disagree on the details of optimal levels for consumption; however, most agree protein should constitute 10–20 percent of your daily intake, carbohydrates 55–65 percent, and fat may supply 20–30 percent. Much of this depends on your individual needs and metabolic characteristics.

Fat intake is commonly very high in dancers. Researchers have reported that fat consumption for female dancers in prominent ballet companies accounts for up to 50 percent of their diet. Much of this fat intake comes from what dancers perceive to be high-protein foods, such as cheese, which are actually very high in fat.

As for the new, synthetic, low-calorie fat substitutes about to come on the market; remember, sugar substitutes have been in use for years and there hasn't exactly been a concomitant net weight loss in American consumers. In terms of weight loss and health, no one knows what the effects of such fat substitutes will be.

10. If you have eaten a normal meal within the last two or three hours, any desire to eat is purely psychological.

While certainly some eating behavior is linked to emotions, the research pendulum has swung across the emotional-physiological gamut in recent years. Psychologists used to approach overweight individuals as primarily having some sort of neurotic disturbance; however, physiologists have illuminated many metabolic changes that influence eating behavior far beyond our psychological control. These physiologic influences were actually established years ago by Ancel Keys, who studied 36 conscientious objectors during World War II in a series of well-planned dietary experiments. In essence, the men ate as they pleased for about 12 weeks to get a baseline caloric intake and body weight. For the following 168 days, the men were put on a 1,600 calorie/day diet, about half their normal intake.

While the expected weight loss (along with lethargy and irritability) ensued, some unexpected results also occurred. The men became obsessed with food and reported that they often fantasized about becoming cooks, waiters, and restaurant owners following the experiment. During the diet period, it was common for them to spend their evenings talking about elaborate culinary concoctions they wanted to cook and extravagant meals they wanted to eat. When the reduced-diet portion of the experiment ended and the men went back to consuming a normal number of calories, they reported that they were still almost constantly hungry and felt unable to get enough food. As they began to regain the lost weight, their body composition changed as well. Abdominal measurements became larger than baseline, indicating that a greater portion of their regained weight was fat. For about half the men, it took nearly three months for them to feel that their interest in food had returned to normal. For others, it took up to a year.

Many conclusions have been derived from this now famous experiment, which has been augmented by other more recent studies. Among other things, this study convinced scientists that when the body is deprived of food, it calls upon every psychological and physiological mechanism at its disposal to drive itself to eat. Although this does not rule out emotional factors in eating behavior, it does put them in perspective. So, if you have ever guiltily lamented over your food obsessions or binges following a diet as being indicative of some slothful personality disorder, consider that you're up against a formidable opponent: your own body's survival mechanisms.

Special Considerations for Dancers

Our first dance science class used to end with this last example until it became obvious how depressed all this made the students. "There's just nothing you can do and win, is there?" they would sigh. While that was *hardly* the case, it was clear that it was unwise to make the students wait until the next class period to hear the other side of the story. The fact is, researchers in weight control have made tremendous strides in recent years and there are more workable methods than ever for aiding the dancer in controlling body composition.

There are a number of characteristics unique to dancers that affect how they should approach weight control. Because these issues will affect how you use the guidelines in this book, we'll state them now and follow up on them later:

1. Unlike athletes who have specific seasons for which they must be in peak condition, dancers have to maintain performance levels of conditioning all year round. This makes it particularly difficult both physiologically and psychologically because there is rarely the feeling that one can "let-up" within the dance regimen. It is for this reason that a diet and exercise plan for dancers must be one that can be sustained throughout the year.

2. Another unique feature of dancers is that most of them are hardly overweight to begin with. In fact, many dancers have what are considered to be normal or below normal body weights, but still do not meet the aesthetic standards demanded by dance. Many dancers must strive for that "ultra" look, which is extremely demanding physically and mentally.

3. The demands of dance training limit how much exercise outside of dance can be done. This is not only because of the fatigue factor and risk of injury, but also because of possible interference with the speed and quickness needed in dance. Another problem is the type of body shape that is developed through certain exercise regimens, which may not fit the classic mold of dance, particularly in ballet. This does not mean exercise to enhance weight loss should not be used by dancers; however, it does mean that the issues above must be considered.

4. Many dancers start their careers at early ages and some are performing professionally by the age of 16. Because the budding of a professional career often coincides with the growth years, it is critical that certain growth processes not be overly sacrificed. It is at this point that one should appreciate the differences between optimal health and optimal performance—the two are not the same. A young girl dieting to try to meet an interested company's weight standards may not be setting a good foundation for her future physiologic and musculoskeletal health; however, her efforts may result in a professional contract. On the other hand, if the dieting becomes excessive, her immediate health may be sacrificed, leaving her unable to pursue dance at all. The dancer must always consider the balance between achieving her goals for dance and maintaining the body that enables her to dance.

These issues will come up again in discussing specific guidelines for nutrition, exercise, and weight control for the performing dancer. Throughout this book we will focus on how to best achieve the necessary balance between maintaining a low body weight for dance and maintaining a healthy body to keep you dancing.

Chapter II   Foundations of Weight Control for Dancers

Diet, Nutrition, and Exercise: Their Combined Effect

No dancer would presume to understand a piece of choreography without considering the intent, movement, music, costuming, and production. Similarly, weight control must be approached through the interrelation of caloric intake, nutritional value, energy output, and psychological factors. A major theme in this book will be how what you consume is converted into energy and how that energy consumption is affected not only by *how much* you eat and *how much* you exercise, but also *the kind* of food you eat and *the kind* of exercise you do. We will discuss the effects of emotions in Chapter 9.

Let's first discuss the individual components of diet, nutrition, and exercise, and set forth some definitions.

DIET: WHAT IS A CALORIE?

When you think "diet," you usually think of calories. A calorie is a standard unit for measuring heat, specifically the amount of heat required to raise the temperature of one gram of water 1° Celsius (C). A kilocalorie (kcal) is the amount of heat necessary to raise one kilogram (kg) of water 1° C. Even though people use the word "calorie" when referring to the content of cheesecake and what you have to do to burn it off, the correct term is "kilocalorie" (abbreviated kcal). (Kcal and calorie are often used interchangeably in diet publications.) Kcals, then, are the measure of energy provided by food to fuel the body.

So, for every kcal you ingest you must generate enough heat to raise one kg of water by 1° C in order to consume the energy provided by that kcal. If you do not generate that amount of heat, that kcal is converted to fat. In the simplest terms, the more heat one generates, the more calories are burned. People who are said to have a "fast" metabolism are simply those whose bodies generate more heat. Thus, in order to lose weight, it is to the dancer's advantage to look for ways to increase the heat generating capacity of the body.

Although the notion of "calories-in-equals-calories-out" in weight loss theory has a certain technical validity, *the way* the body metabolizes food plays a much greater role than previously thought. That is, you can't just measure what a person eats and estimate the caloric expenditure to arrive at how much weight should be lost. The rate of metabolism must also be considered, just as you wouldn't estimate how long you should bake a cake without considering the oven temperature. The body's biochemical processes can serve to regulate your body's "oven temperature," and can be influenced by nutrition and exercise to make sure things stay "hot."

NUTRITION

Nutrition is not the same as caloric intake, as anyone knows who has watched a teenager down nothing but Ding-Dongs for lunch. For the purposes of this book we will define nutrition as those elements of food intake that ensure maintenance of bodily functions and promote optimal performance. Although caloric intake is part of nutrition, it is the quality of that caloric intake that will make up our focus on nutrition.

Good nutrition often gets nothing more than lip-service from those wanting to lose weight because if a choice were demanded between balanced nutrition and losing five pounds, we can guess which one would win. However, nutrition involves much more than the four food groups that bored us all in grade school. In fact, the nutritional content of the foods you choose can have as much to do with weight loss as the calories that you consume.

Nutrition involves dietary balance of protein, carbohydrate, and fat, as well as vitamins and minerals. The balance and nutrient density of your diet can also influence your metabolic rate and how your body responds to exercise, as we will see in the following analysis of fuel sources and exercise.

EXERCISE: HARDER IS NOT NECESSARILY BETTER

Lifting weights is exercise. Dancing an allegro variation is exercise. Running three miles is exercise, and so is walking five miles. All these activities can be described as exercise, yet they all use the body's energy sources in different ways. Weight-lifting requires short bursts of very high energy. The energy requirements for allegro are longer, perhaps a minute or two, and although the energy output is also high, it is not as concentrated as that involved in weight lifting. Running three miles may burn the same number of calories as walking five miles, but the run is fueled primarily by sugar stores, whereas the walk uses fat stores as its primary fuel source.

We could simply end our discussion of fuel sources in exercise here; however, we would have to leave out some important information, although it is rather dense and technical. We have found that most dancers are interested in how the body works on every level, and are willing to wade through some tough terminology in order to understand the nitty-gritty. Therefore, what follows is a more precise, although simplified, explanation of these concepts using straight physiologic terminology. So, warning on the Greek, and if it all sounds confusing the first time through, that's only because it is.*

The main sources of energy in the body are phosphorus, glucose, and fat (see Figure 2.1). All energy in the body is directly supplied by the breakdown of the molecule *adenosine triphosphate* (ATP), but the aforementioned "substrates," or fuel sources, all serve to produce ATP via different processes. So, phosphorus, glucose, and fat can all be converted into ATP, which is then converted into energy. (Protein can also be used as an indirect energy source under special circumstances that will be discussed later.)

Phosphorus is the "quick-and-dirty" fuel source when the body needs an extraordinary amount of energy in a very short time frame. The energy to lift a heavy object is supplied primarily through the system in which a phosphorus and creatine molecule (phosphocreatine) forms an ATP

*For more information on diet physiology, consult the bibliography.

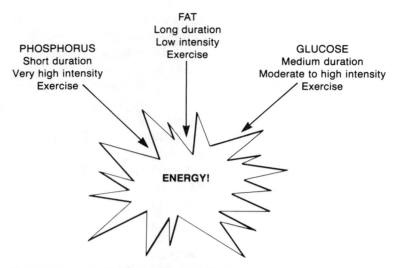

Figure 2.1. Fuel Sources for Energy Production

molecule. The energy supply is high, but the length of time it can be sustained is extremely short: less than a few seconds.

Glucose produces ATP for intermediate periods of energy demand, although the preferential use of glucose depends on the duration and intensity of the activity. In a short period of activity, such as an allegro, energy is supplied through a mechanism known as *anaerobic glycolysis*. This literally means cutting-off *(lysis)* of a unit of a glycogen molecule (glycogen is just a bunch of glucoses strung together) and metabolized without oxygen *(anaerobic)*. Of course there's always oxygen in your body, but in order for this process to run as quickly as it needs to, the direct use of oxygen to form ATP is bypassed. Instead of using oxygen molecules for the key biochemical processes that make ATP, the body forms lactic acid.

Glucose is also the major fuel source for an activity like medium-distance running, but here's where things get murky. The type of fuel source that predominates at this point depends on how hard you run, how far, and what kind of shape you're in. If you are in average running condition and run three miles in 20 minutes, the main substrate will be glucose broken down into ATP via *aerobic glycolysis*. The difference between *anaerobic* and *aerobic* glycolysis is that in aerobic glycolysis oxygen is used as the key factor in maintaining the generation of ATP, whereas in anaerobic glycolysis lactic acid is used (indirectly) to maintain the generation of ATP. Aerobic glycolysis is a slower process than anaerobic glycolysis and predominates when the intensity of the exercise is not as great. Glucose is the fuel source for both processes, but it is used to make ATP via different metabolic pathways.

Finally, fat is used as a source of fuel in a process called *aerobic lipolysis* (*lipo* meaning lipid or fat). Fat molecules are big and difficult to break down, so the formation of ATP from fat is very slow. There are four factors that determine if fat is used as the primary substrate: (a) energy demand; (b) duration of the activity; (c) condition of the person; and (d) nutritional status of the person.

For factor (a), if the energy demands are too great, the slow lipolysis process can't keep pace and the body must use aerobic glycolysis. So, the type of exercise that promotes fat burning is low- to moderate-intensity, which is indicated by how fast your heart beats during the activity.

Duration, factor (b), is also important because the body's ability to burn fat during exercise takes a while to get "geared up." This has a lot to do with hormonal releases in response to intensity and duration of exercise. In general, it takes about 30 minutes of low- to moderate-intensity exercise for the metabolic reactions involving lipolysis to predominate. This is why fat burning exercise is termed endurance exercise.

Factor (c), conditioning, comes into play according to how fit you are for endurance exercise. If you are well-conditioned, your body burns fat more readily than if you are not. So, a well-conditioned person will burn more fat sooner than someone poorly conditioned when engaged in a bout of endurance exercise. However, the conditioning must be *specific* to endurance exercise; for example, a well-conditioned dancer is not the same as a well-conditioned endurance athlete.

Nutritional status, factor (d), has to do with how long prior to exercise you have eaten and what you ate. If you consume a food that is mostly glucose (or carbohydrate) less than an hour before exercising, your body will use that glucose as its fuel source rather than begin to recruit fat stores. You will still burn all or some of the calories provided by the food you just ate, but the exercise session will not burn as much fat.

So, if you were to walk at a moderate but steady pace for at least 30 minutes, were in good condition for endurance exercise, and had not eaten any sugar or starches within the hour prior to exercise, the primary source of fuel would be fat.

Having said all that, be aware that none of these processes occur in an all-or-none fashion. It is really a matter of degree, and these categories are based on the fuel source that is used *predominantly* during the described activities. In fact, as you sit reading this book, you are engaged in aerobic glycolysis and aerobic lipolysis because even at rest, you are producing energy just by being alive.

Protein is not used as a direct fuel source. Protein is primarily needed to maintain, build, or rebuild muscle and bone, but it does not provide energy for exercise to any extent. The only way protein is ever used as an energy source to any significant degree is during starvation. Even then, protein is an indirect fuel source because it must first be converted to glucose before it can be used.

If all this seems like a jumble of technicalities, don't be dismayed. Look over Figure 2.2 and remember that it is the gist of these concepts that is important, not the detail.

We can now see that when it comes to weight control, the *kind* of exercise you do is as important as *how much* you do, and that working harder is not necessarily better for promoting fat loss. We can also see that what you eat and when you eat can have an effect on how much fat or glucose you burn for energy. So truly, we cannot separate diet, nutrition, and exercise in our weight control efforts.

The kind of activity involved in dance uses primarily anaerobic glycolysis—that is, repeated short bursts of intense activity as opposed to long periods of sustained, moderate activity. As we have just seen, it is the latter that promotes fat utilization. This is obviously a dilemma for dancers: dance aesthetics require a lean body, but dance activity does not promote fat loss.

Fortunately, this does not mean dancers are stuck. Choos-

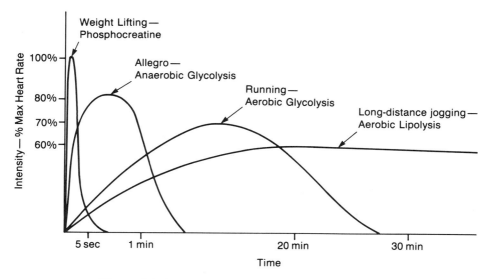

Figure 2.2. Intensity of Activity Over Time: Relationship to Metabolic Energy Production

ing the right kind of exercise program to complement your dietary efforts and your dance training can lead to the achievement of a lithe and lean body. These exercise and diet choices will be further discussed in Chapters 6 and 8.

Metabolism: Fast versus Slow

Diet, nutrition, and exercise work together to affect metabolic rate. We often refer to having a slow or fast metabolism, but what does this really mean? Metabolism comes from the Greek word *metaballein,* meaning to change or alter. In a general sense, metabolism may be defined as tissue change. For our purposes, we will focus on the specific aspects of the breakdown of food and production of energy.

When someone is said to have a "fast" metabolism, the reference is usually to being able to eat a lot and not gain weight. Basically such a person produces a lot of excess heat and thus burns up extra calories. A person with a "slow" metabolism does not generate or "waste" many calories as heat but is good at storing excess calories as fat. For weight/fat-loss purposes, you want to be good at "wasting" calories, which is done by producing excess heat.

Metabolism takes place in every cell in the body, but we're going to talk primarily about metabolism in muscle cells because they generate the need for extra energy. The muscle cell is actually quite complex, but the two elements we're concerned with are those that burn glucose very fast (the anaerobic functions) and those that burn glucose and/or fat more slowly (the aerobic functions).

The anaerobic elements of the cell are geared toward the fast breakdown of glucose. These anaerobic elements increase and become stronger in response to high-intensity, short-duration training such as dance. The slow aerobic parts of the cell become stronger and increase in number with endurance training.

Because you can only break down fats in the slow aerobic part of the cell, the endurance-trained person is going to be much better at breaking down fats for fuel than the dancer or other anaerobically trained person. Although a dancer will never be able to burn fat for most kinds of ballet or traditional modern dancing, you can increase your fat-burning capacity by augmenting your dancing with endurance exercise. (A few modern choreographers do work in a kind of dance-endurance style.) Endurance exercise not only burns calories while you're performing it, it also helps keep your metabolic rate higher overall than if you didn't exercise.

However, if a dancer's primary activity is anaerobic, wouldn't it be detrimental to a dancer to train aerobically? If the aerobic training becomes excessive compared to the amount of anaerobic training, yes, the dancer might compromise his or her ability to perform high-intensity dance activities. But we are not talking about training exclusively in an endurance fashion; one can augment dance training with endurance exercise for the specific purpose of promoting fat loss without interfering with dance technique, if it is done properly.

THE DOWNS AND UPS OF STARVATION

Because all dieting is basically a form of intentional starvation, it is important to understand the metabolic adjustments that take place during extreme food deprivation. Although we will include some biochemical facts and figures, it is only so that ultimately the big picture concerning weight control will be more clear. When consuming a very low-carbohydrate diet (less than 60 grams of carbohydrate a day), the body reacts almost as if it had no food at all, so for our purposes we will refer to the two situations simultaneously.

A typical man weighing 150 lb has fuel reserves of about 1,600 kcal in glycogen, 24,000 kcal in usable protein, and 135,000 kcal in fat. The glucose requirement of the brain in a typical adult is about 120 grams per day, which accounts for most of the 160 grams of glucose needed by the whole body. There are about 20 grams of glucose stored in body fluids and about 190 grams stored as glycogen. These direct glucose reserves are sufficient to meet the body and brain's glucose needs for about 24 hours.

In starvation, the body's first priority is to provide sufficient glucose to the brain and other tissues, such as red blood cells, that are absolutely dependent on this fuel. Fat *cannot* be converted into glucose to any appreciable extent, so sustaining the brain and red blood cells during the first few days of starvation must be accomplished by converting protein into glucose. Direct conversion of protein into ATP for energy cannot take place; protein must first be converted into glucose and then converted to ATP. The process of converting protein to glucose is known as *gluconeogenesis* (new generation of glucose).

Gluconeogenesis affects fat breakdown because it depletes the supply of an important element necessary for the complete breakdown of fats. Because of this, fats undergo only partial breakdown, which results in the formation of *ketones*. Ketones are then released into the blood and have important metabolic ramifications.

During the first three days of starvation, the body's first priority is to break down protein (first muscle and then liver tissue) to supply the brain and red blood cells with glucose. However, the body's second priority in starvation is to *preserve* its liver and muscle tissue. Therefore, after about three days of starvation, the large amounts of ketones that have been formed as a result of gluconeogenesis become about a third of the fuel source for the brain. This adaptation to ketones as a fuel source is a process that develops in response to at least three days of starvation or carbohydrate depletion.

After several weeks of starvation, ketones become the major fuel source for the brain. By that time, only about 40 grams of glucose is needed per day for the brain, compared with about 120 grams the first day of starvation. Because ketones are now used as a replacement for glucose, much less muscle tissue is broken down than in the first days of starvation. After three days of starvation, the body breaks down about 75 grams of protein per day for fuel, compared to only 20 grams per day after several weeks of starvation. Fuel sources used after three days of starvation vs. 40 days are depicted in Table 2.1.

As we mentioned in Chapter 1, starvation may look like a great way to lose weight. In fact, for some obese individuals, medically supervised starvation or liquid-protein supplement fasting is sometimes necessary. A great deal of media attention has focused on liquid-diet programs such as Opti-Fast, which was followed by celebrity Oprah Winfrey. However, just so there are no misunderstandings, such plans are usually available only to medically obese individuals and come at no small price.

The average cost for the OptiFast program is $3,300, which includes medical supervision during the fast and behavioral, nutritional, and exercise counseling. Those accepted into the program have an average of 60 pounds to lose. The program consists of a completely liquid diet for twelve weeks, followed by a gradual refeeding of solid food, which lasts for six weeks. According to Rachel Dawson, former dancer and present director of an OptiFast program in Salt Lake City, the most important aspects of the program are the behavioral and nutritional counseling along with aerobic exercise, which are fundamental to the success of the plan. Programs such as OptiFast make no guarantees, and, in fact, there is a significant drop-out and failure rate. However, for those whose obesity is seriously threatening their health, such programs can truly be a life-saver.. But unless you are a dancer who is more than 50 pounds over normal weight, such regimens are simply not appropriate.

Table 2.1. Fuel Sources in Starvation

Fuel Exchanges and Consumption	Amount Formed or Consumed in 24 Hours (Grams)	
	3rd day	40th day
Fuel use by brain		
Glucose	100	40
Ketones	50	100
All other use of glucose	50	40
Fuel mobilization		
Fat breakdown	180	180
Muscle-protein breakdown	75	20
Fuel output by liver		
Glucose	150	80
Ketones	150	150

From *Biochemistry*, 3rd ed. by Lubert Stryer. Copyright © 1975, 1981, 1988. Reprinted with the permission of W. H. Freeman and Company.

For most anyone who has ever tried a starvation diet, it is clear that it is what happens *after* starvation that leads to so many failures. In starvation, even though the numbers on your scale may initally go down, afterwards they too often rise back up—and up and up.

When refeeding starts, the body kicks in every mechanism at its disposal to restore its glycogen stores and *fat* deposits first. The first weight regained upon refeeding is water (for the storage of glycogen), and then the body points all its instincts in the direction of fat restoration. As found in studies of starvation and refeeding, all psychological and physiological mechanisms join forces to drive the person to eat enough to rebuild depleted fat stores.

This is one reason why starvation dieters tend to regain their lost weight with a greater proportion of the regained weight as fat. This vicious cycle continues with many unfortunate dieters ending up fatter than when they started dieting. This is also why many diet experts feel that slow changes in body composition will be more likely to result in permanent changes. As the body has time to adjust to its decreased fat stores, the mechanisms that lead toward binging are less likely to surface.

Coordinate Your Efforts

Dancers often ask, "Why don't I lose weight when I eat so little?" Now that we have more closely examined the roles of diet, nutrition, and exercise, it should be clear that these factors work in concert as they apply to your weight control efforts. In large part, these cofactors are why "the chocolate cake diet" and other gems of the fad-diet industry simply do not work. The interaction of metabolic rate and diet is also why many dancers can eat very little and still not lose weight. The more one cuts calories, the more efficient the body becomes at conserving energy, which is why many dancers don't lose weight despite a chronically low caloric intake.

However, endurance training can serve to maintain or even increase metabolic rate while dieting. Such exercise helps maintain muscle stores, which are the generators of energy and ultimately serve to burn more fat. We will discuss these effects in later chapters, but first we will examine the specifics of body composition, that is, how much of you is muscle and how much is fat.

Chapter III   Body Composition

Muscle Weight vs. Fat Weight

In Chapter 2, we discussed burning fat vs. burning glucose. All this ties into our ultimate goal of attaining the type of body that is aesthetically and physically suitable for dance. Just as there are different kinds of exercise, so are there different kinds of weight loss, with each kind resulting in different changes in body composition.

Body composition involves how much of your total body weight consists of muscle, bone, fat, water, and "other stuff" (ash, minerals, etc.). Every person is made up of a certain proportion of these elements. Two people can weigh the same but have different proportions of fat and muscle, which are the two variables we are most concerned with here. The proportion of fat is usually described as a percentage of total body weight and is known as "percent body fat." The proportion of muscle, bone, and other elements is usually described in total pounds and is known as "lean body weight" or "lean body mass."

To illustrate how this works, let's take two people who are the same height, 5'7, and weight, 120 lb. One person has 13 percent body fat and the other has 21 percent body fat. When we work out the percentages in terms of fat and muscle weight, we get the results listed in the Table 3.1.

Now, consider that the average pound of fat takes up about 31 cubic inches of space and the average pound of lean tissue takes up 25 cubic inches of space.* Multiply 15.6 lb of fat by 31 to get 484 cubic inches and 25.2 lb of fat by 31 to get 781 cubic inches, and do the same with lean body weight multiplied by 25. The differences in volume between a 13 percent and 21 percent fat person are listed in Table 3.2.

When we add up total body cubic inches we find that the 13 percent body fat person has almost 60 cubic inches less "body" than the 21 percent person, yet they weigh exactly

*Fat density = .90 grams per cubic cm. Lean tissue density = 1. 10 grams per cubic cm (Katch & McArdle, 1983, p. 110).

Table 3.1. Body Composition for Different Proportions of Fat

	13% Body Fat	21% Body Fat
Total Weight (lb)	120.0	120.0
Height (in.)	67.0	67.0
Fat (lb)	15.6	25.2
Lean Body Wt (lb)	104.4	94.8

the same and are the same height. Therefore, by lowering your percent body fat, you can reduce your body size even if you don't lose weight. This is simply because lean body mass is more dense (more compact) than fat.

When you go on a starvation or very low-calorie diet, the majority of the initial weight-loss comes from water and muscle. During the first seven to ten days of such a diet, about 85 percent of the weight lost is from water (due to the loss of glycogen) and muscle (due to the use of protein tissue for gluconeogenesis). Therefore, short-term "crash" diets are not effective for losing appreciable amounts of fat.

Another phenomenon that adds insult to injury is from where on your body you lose most of the muscle. When the body must use muscle for fuel, it will burn the muscle tissue that is least used first. In dancers, who work heavily with their legs and hips, muscle is first lost from the shoulders, face, and upper body. Of course dancers use their upper bodies, but not with the same resistance that they use their legs and hips. So, the upper torso and arms thin out while the lower body remains intact, thus accentuating the unwanted "thunder thighs" look.

We can see that it is important to assess not just how much you weigh, but also what makes up that weight. Although

Table 3.2. Volumetric Differences in Body Composition

	13% Body Fat	21% Body Fat
Cubic inches fat	484	781
Cubic inches lean mass	2,610	2,370
Total cubic inches	3,094	3,151
Difference = 57 total cubic inches		

there is much variability in assessing body composition, there have been a number of studies conducted on dancers to determine just what is the average dancer's percent body fat.

Dancers' Body Composition: Research Results

What is the average percent body fat level for a female dancer? Professional ballet dancers have been studied most frequently in this area, with average values for females ranging from about 11–17 percent body fat, depending on the study (Calabrese et al., 1983a; Chmelar et al., 1988a; Cohen et al., 1985; Kirkendall & Calabrese, 1983; Micheli et al., 1984; Ryan & Stephens, 1989; White, 1982). In our study of body composition in different styles and levels of female dancers (Chmelar et al., 1988a), we measured the percent fat values listed in Table 3.3.

These values mean that among 21 advanced-level, university ballet and modern dancers, there was virtually no difference in the average percent body fat, that is, between 14.2 and 14.7 percent. This shows that most of these dancers, who all participated in student performing groups, maintained a relatively low percent body fat. The professional dancers, both ballet and modern, were slightly leaner on average, although not significantly so. The professional modern dancers in this study were very lean, with an average of 12.2 percent body fat.

Table 3.3. Body Composition in Different Levels and Styles of Female Dancers (Chmelar et al., 1988)

	Height (in.)	Weight (lb)	Percent Fat	Percent Fat Range
University				
Ballet (n = 10)	65.3 ± 2.0*	117.7 ± 10.4	14.2 ± 3.2	9.6–20.5
Modern (n = 11)	64.5 ± 1.4	119.8 ± 9.3	14.7 ± 3.4	10.9–23.6
Professional				
Ballet (n = 9)	65.9 ± 2.5	119.4 ± 9.3	14.1 ± 1.9	11.2–17.6
Modern (n = 9)	63.7 ± 2.9	114.9 ± 13.0	12.2 ± 2.1	9.6–16.1

*Mean ± Standard Deviation.

Figure 3.1a shows a graph of what various dance researchers have found for percent body fat among female professional, preprofessional, and university dancers in comparison to those for selected female athletes. When compared to most female athletes, professional dancers are quite lean.

As for male dancers (Figure 3.1b), Cohen et al. (1985) found an average of 7.8 percent fat with a range of 5.7 to 10.4 percent (professional ballet). In our unpublished pilot study of male professional modern dancers (Chmelar & Smith, 1984 unpublished), we found an average of 7.4 percent fat, while Haviland's (1978) college-male modern dancers had an average of 7.9 percent fat. Ryan and Stephens (1989), however, reported an average of 13 percent fat for Ballet West male dancers, and 11.7 percent for Ballet West advanced male students. This discrepancy between the results of Ryan and Stephens and the other dance researchers is most likely due to the fact that different skinfold equations were used in measuring percent fat.

The above information simply reflects the *average* results from research on percent body fat in dancers. Later in this chapter, we will provide guidelines on percent fat for professional and university dancers.

Methods for Estimating Percent Body Fat

In assessing your own weight modification goals, knowing your particular body composition can help you design the best weight control approach. Also, because most university dance programs and professional companies have weight guidelines, the directors involved should consider adding measurements of body composition to their programs. There are a number of methods for measuring percent body fat, but the following are most often used:

1. *Hydrostatic (underwater) weighing.* Weighing a body underwater gives an estimation of the person's body *density*, which is mass-per-unit volume. The greater your density, the less fat you have.

Hydrostatic weighing requires specialized equipment, not the least of which is a pool or tank large enough for complete submersion. This makes the technique impractical, plus it is a cumbersome and time-consuming undertaking. However,

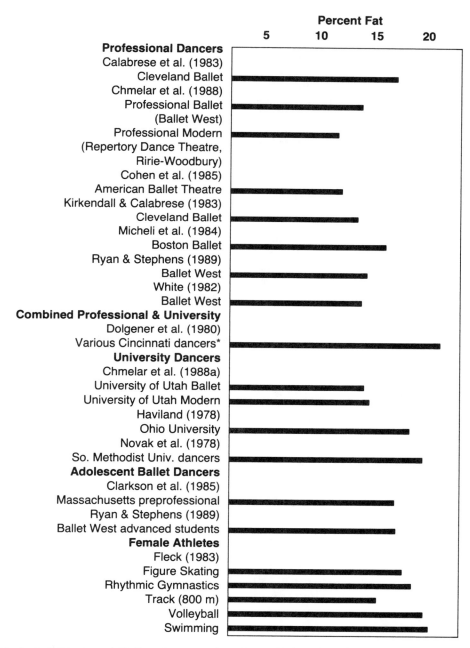

*Included Cincinnati Ballet, dance majors from University of Cincinnati College Conservatory of Music, and professional modern companies in Cincinnati.

Figure 3.1a. Results of Research on Body Composition for Female Dancers and Athletes

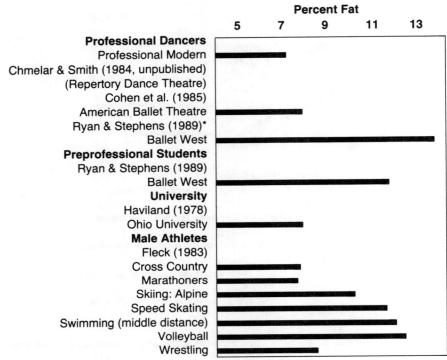

*Differences in skinfold equations can account for significant variations in results. Ryan & Stephens used the Durnin formula whereas the other dance researchers used the Jackson & Pollock formula.

Figure 3.1b. Results of Research on Body Composition for Male Dancers and Athletes

of all indirect assessment methods available to the general public, it is the most accurate *if conducted by qualified personnel*.

2. *Bioelectrical Impedance.* This method works on the principle of electrical impedance, which simply means how well an electrical current is conducted through a given medium. Water is a good conductor for electricity, so the more water in a substance the better electricity is conducted. Since muscle is largely water, the theory behind using electrical impedance for estimation of body composition is that the greater the proportion of muscle, the greater the conductivity. Once muscle mass is estimated, percent fat can be derived from knowing the person's total weight.

Bioelectrical impedance requires specialized equipment, which runs about $5,000, although it is very easy and convenient to use. Unfortunately, the results can be skewed by a number of variables: how much water the person usually drinks, body temperature, differences in skin conductivity, and so on. So, in order to be accurate, this method must be used under strictly controlled conditions, which is a problem when testing dancers.

3. *Skinfold-girth measurements.* Approximately 50 percent of the fat in your body is subcutaneous or "under the skin." The other 50 percent is visceral, that is, surrounding the abdominal organs. Therefore, if we measure the fat just under the skin by doing what is essentially a "pinch" test, we can estimate the person's percent body fat.

This method requires a metric tape measure, skinfold calipers (which run anywhere from a few dollars to $150), and someone well-trained in the technique and calculations involved. There are computerized calipers available which calculate percent fat for you; however, they run about $500 and you're limited to using the equations programmed into the device, most of which are inappropriate for dancers.

Naturally, different body fat standards must be used for different groups, but another important consideration in using skinfold methods is that the *equation* also be specific to the population being tested. That is, not only do you need to use different standards when comparing percent fat in football players versus dancers, you should also use an estimation equation that is specifically designed for dancers. Skinfold equations are designed by correlating the results of hydrostatic weighing with specific skinfold and girth measurements for a given group of people. Therefore, if you are going to use skinfold measurements to test percent body fat in dancers, you should use an equation that was developed on a group with similar physical characteristics. Also, you cannot use the same equation to estimate percent fat in female dancers as male dancers.

SKINFOLD-GIRTH METHOD FOR FEMALE DANCERS

Unfortunately, no one has yet done a study that we know of specifically on a skinfold-girth equation for estimating percent fat in dancers. However, there is a very good equation, developed on gymnasts, which has proven to be appropriate for most female dancers (Sinning, 1978). This equation involves the following measurements:

A. Circumference of the neck (mid-neck) in centimeters (cm).
B. Supra-iliac skinfold, two inches above the right anterior superior iliac spine, taken obliquely (on a diagonal), in millimeters (mm).
C. Abdominal skinfold, just to the right (about 2 cm) of the umbilicus (navel), in mm.

These values, A, B, and C, are then plugged into the following equation:

1.02462 + (0.002024 × A) − (0.001435 × B) − (0.001039 × C) = Density

The value for Density is then used in the following equation (Siri equation, see Fox & Mathews, 1981, p. 526):

[(4.95 ÷ Density) − 4.50] × 100 = Percent Body Fat

For all our fellow math cowards, do not be put off by the six decimal place figures. These equations are not difficult, they just require a lot of number punching. Let's go through an example:
A. *31.5 cm* − circumference of the neck
B. *6.0 mm* − supra-iliac skinfold
C. *7.5 mm* − abdominal skinfold

1.02462 + (0.002024 × *31.5 cm*) − (0.001435 × *6.0 mm*) − (0.001039 × *7.5 mm*) = 1.0719735
[(4.95/1.0719735) − 4.50] × 100 = 11.7654 = *11.8 Percent Body Fat*

If you didn't get the answers above for Density and Percent Body Fat, check your math with the bracket solutions shown below:

1.02462 + (0.063756) − (0.00861) − (0.0077925) = 1.0719735
[(4.61765) − 4.50] × 100 = 11.7654 = 11.76 percent Body Fat

As you can see, we don't actually use the person's body weight in these equations. That is because we are simply trying to determine body density and then calculating percent fat. If we wanted to know how many pounds of fat this person has we would need to know her total weight, which happens to be 124.3 lb. If we multiply 124.3 by the decimal value for percent fat, .118, we get our answer: 14.7 pounds of fat. To get lean body weight, simply subtract 14.7 from 124.3, which equals 109.6 pounds, Therefore:

Total Weight × [Percent Fat/100] = Fat Weight
Total Weight − Fat Weight = Lean Body Weight

SKINFOLD METHOD FOR BODY FAT ESTIMATION IN MALE DANCERS

Three skinfold sites are used in this method, which was developed on light-to medium-build athletic males (Boscardin et al., 1988):

1. Triceps: A vertical fold is taken on the back of the upper arm over the triceps, midway between the elbow and the acromion of the shoulder (outermost bony landmark of the shoulder girdle). The arm should hang naturally as the skinfold is measured.

2. Abdominals: A vertical fold is taken just to the right side of the umbilicus (navel).

3. Pectorals: A diagonal fold is taken just below the crease at the front of the armpit.

The following equation is then used to estimate percent fat:

Percent Fat = 6.036 + .446(T) + .279(A) − .486(P)

In the above formula, T represents the triceps skinfold in mm, A the abdominal skinfold, and P the pectoral skinfold.

GUIDELINES FOR USING SKINFOLD-GIRTH MEASUREMENTS

If you decide to use a skinfold-girth method, be sure to follow these guidelines:

1. Carefully determine each site from the correct anatomical landmark and then mark it with water-soluble marker so that your measurements are consistent.

2. When doing a skinfold measurement, maintain the fold between your thumb and forefinger while you take the measurement with the calipers. *Do not let go* once the calipers have grasped the skinfold. If you have difficulty grasping the skinfold, have the subject tense the muscle, then grasp the skinfold and have the subject relax while the measurement is taken.

3. For girth measurements, a steel tape is best since it doesn't stretch like cloth or plastic.

4. Take three measurements at each site to ensure accuracy. Record each measurement immediately after taking it.

5. Once three measurements have been taken, use the average of the two values with the least variability for your final value. For example, given the values 32.4, 31.4, and 31.6 you should average 31.4 and 31.6 for your most accurate value. Why? Because chances are that 32.4 is subject to the most error and would skew your final value toward that error if you used it in averaging all three numbers. If all three values are equally distributed, such as 31.5, 31.6, and 31.4, then average all three.

6. When doing the calculations, do not round off until you get to the final value for percent fat. Small differences in the initial calculation for density can result in a large error in the percent fat value.

7. As much as possible have *one* trained person take these measurements. This person should also practice on a number of dancers over a period of days to ensure that they are consistent before actually measuring for the record.

8. Make note of where the female subject is in her menstrual cycle at the time of testing. If the test is scheduled within three days of the onset of her period, the results may be skewed due to premenstrual water retention. If this is the case, be sure to retest the subject at another time.

9. IMPORTANT NOTE! Skinfold measurements have been shown to be of no value in predicting changes in body composition following weight loss. Why? Because weight loss occurs first in internal abdominal fat, which would not be detected by skinfold measurements. The fact of the matter is that no single body composition method has yet been shown to be reliable enough to assess changes due to weight loss, especially when they are on the magnitude of 5 or 10 lb. However, these methods can certainly be used to give dancers a good idea of what their percent body fat is and what they would like it to be. (See Tables 3.5 and 3.6 for guidelines on percent fat for female and male dancers.)

To evaluate someone's weight loss progress, you should also consider changes in total weight and changes in overall girth measurements, which we will discuss in the next section.

GIRTH MEASUREMENTS

Because we are limited in our ability to accurately assess changes in body composition with skinfold techniques, using girth measurements can help determine a person's progress. Girths can be best used as a relative measure to assess changes in body proportions.

The following sites should be measured (all values in cm):

1. Upper arm: Midway between the elbow and lateral bony prominence of the shoulder (acromion). Elbow should be extended with arm abducted to 90° in the coronal plane (straight to the side at shoulder level).
2. Bust (women)/Chest (men): At point of maximum girth.
3. Waist: At point of minimum girth, about one inch above the navel.
4. Hips: At maximum girth with feet parallel and hip width apart.
5. Mid-thigh: For most dancers, 15–16 cm above the superior border of the patella (kneecap). May be more or less for extremely tall or short dancers. Note distance in recording data.

Dolgener et al. (1980) have looked at these and other indices of body build among female ballet and modern dancers. These measurements, listed in Table 3.4, were taken on a combined population of professional and university performers.

Table 3.4. Girth Measurements for Female Dancers (Dolgener et al., 1980)

	Ballet	Modern
Upper Arm (cm)	21.7	23.0
Bust	81.0	81.5
Waist	63.0	62.4
Hips	84.9	88.5
Thigh	50.1	50.5
Height (in.)	64.6	64.5
Weight (lb)	112.4	117.0

Guidelines for Percent Fat in Dancers

As previously discussed, the proportion of fat to lean weight for a dancer of a given total weight and height are ultimately what make up the dancer's aesthetic appearance. In trying to determine your ideal proportions, your height, weight, and percent fat should be considered. Many university dance departments and professional companies have height and weight requirements. However, in order to give a more accurate picture of the dancer's total proportions, guidelines for percent fat and fat weight should also be incorporated.

FEMALE DANCERS: PROFESSIONAL AND UNIVERSITY

Table 3.5 lists typical ranges of body composition based on studies of professional and university *adult* female dancers. Pre-professional adolescent dancers should set their body-fat goals no lower than the high end of the professional range in order to avoid problems with growth and development. The figures for university dancers are higher in order to accommodate the wider range of body-types and career goals in university programs. These values for percent body

Table 3.5. Percent Body Fat Ranges for Professional and University Female Dancers

Height (ft'in.)	Weight (lb)	% Body Fat Professional	Fat Weight (lb)	% Body Fat University	Fat Weight (lb)
4'10	75–85	11–17	8.3–12.8*	17–23	12.8–17.3*
4'11	80–90	11–17	8.8–13.6	17–23	13.6–18.4
5'0	85–95	11–17	9.4–14.5	17–23	14.5–19.6
5'1	90–100	11–17	9.9–15.3	17–23	15.3–20.7
5'2	95–105	11–17	10.5–16.2	17–23	16.2–21.9
5'3	100–111	11–17	11.0–17.0	17–23	17.0–23.0
5'4	105–116	11–17	11.6–17.9	17–23	17.9–24.2
5'5	110–121	11–17	12.1–18.7	17–23	18.7–25.3
5'6	115–127	11–17	12.7–19.6	17–23	19.6–26.5
5'7	120–132	11–17	13.2–20.4	17–23	20.4–27.6
5'8	125–137	11–17	13.8–21.3	17–23	21.3–28.8
5'9	130–144	11–17	14.3–22.1	17–23	22.1–29.9
5'10	135–149	11–17	14.9–23.0	17–23	23.0–31.5
5'11	140–154	11–17	15.4–23.8	17–23	23.8–32.2
6'0	145–160	11–17	16.0–24.7	17–23	24.7–33.4
6'1	150–175	11–17	16.5–25.5	17–23	25.5–34.5

*Maximal fat weight is based on highest percent fat relative to lowest total weight.

fat should not be used as precise cut-off points, but rather they should give dancers, instructors, and company directors a fair idea of what levels of body fat are appropriate relative to height and weight.

MALE DANCERS: PROFESSIONAL AND UNIVERSITY

Overall, few male dancers have the kinds of weight problems that female dancers have, primarily because aesthetic standards for men in dance are closer to the ideal weights of nondance men (as set by insurance companies), whereas standards for women in dance are much lower. Most male dancers are concerned with fine-tuning their proportions through weight training and adjustments in technique. But for those male dancers who do need to make changes in their body composition, Table 3.6 can be used as a guide.

Guidelines for a Body Composition Assessment Program

If your university program or professional company is interested in incorporating body composition assessment into its weight evaluations, the following guidelines should be used in order to ensure accurate and fair application of the results:

1. Schedule the initial assessment for a given year or season approximately two weeks after classes or rehearsals have begun. In order to get good baseline data, you should wait until your dancers have established their routine so that they are at comparable activity levels at the time of testing.

2. Measurements to be taken should include: height, dry weight (be sure the scale is accurately calibrated), girth measurements (see previous section), and those for body composition analysis.

• If skinfold-girth methods are used for body composition, *be sure to follow the guidelines listed on page 35–36.* Two people should be present for the measurements: one to take the measurements and the other to record them.

• If a different method is used, such as hydrostatic weighing, be sure that the person conducting the test is well-qualified. Your best bet is to find someone associated with a university exercise physiology program, although hospital wellness centers may also offer hydrostatic weighing serv-

Table 3.6. Percent Body Fat Ranges for Professional and University Male Dancers

Height (ft'in.)	Weight (lb)	% Body Fat Professional	Fat Weight (lb)	% Body Fat University	Fat Weight (lb)
5'2	110–120	5–11	5.5–12.1	8–13	8.8–14.3
5'3	115–125	5–11	5.8–12.6	8–13	9.2–15.0
5'4	120–130	5–11	6.0–13.2	8–13	9.6–15.6
5'5	125–135	5–11	6.3–13.8	8–13	10.0–16.3
5'6	130–140	5–11	6.5–14.3	8–13	10.4–16.9
5'7	135–146	5–11	6.8–14.8	8–13	10.8–17.6
5'8	140–151	5–11	7.0–15.4	8–13	11.2–18.2
5'9	145–156	5–11	7.3–16.0	8–13	11.6–19.3
5'10	150–162	5–11	7.5–16.5	8–13	12.0–19.5
5'11	155–167	5–11	7.8–17.1	8–13	12.4–20.2
6'0	160–172	5–11	8.0–17.6	8–13	12.8–20.8
6'1	165–177	5–11	8.3–18.2	8–13	13.2–21.5
6'2	170–185	5–11	8.5–18.7	8–13	13.6–22.1
6'3	175–190	5–11	8.8–19.3	8–13	14.0–22.8
6'4	180–195	5–11	9.0–19.8	8–13	14.4–23.4

*Maximal fat weight is based on highest percent fat relative to lowest total weight.

ices. Be wary of health club assessments since very often there is frequent turnover in personnel and a lack of appropriate training. Be sure the person has conducted and analyzed at least 50 such tests.

3. Time of day. If at all possible, these measurements should be taken first thing in the morning before the dancer has had anything to eat or drink. If this is not possible, the next-best time would be just before lunch and if not then, just before dinner. Whatever time is chosen, be sure that the time for any follow-up evaluations is the same.

4. Follow-up testing. General follow-up should be scheduled about 10–12 weeks after the initial test. For most university programs one test at the beginning of the semester or quarter and one at the end should suffice.

If a dancer is found to be significantly above or below the standards of your company or program, follow-up should be designed on an individual basis. For example, Mary Doe is a professional dancer, 63 inches (160 cm) tall, 128 lb, and 18 percent body fat. Her girth measurements are upper arm: 25.4 cm, bust: 88.2 cm, waist: 68.0 cm, hips: 91.1 cm, thigh: 53.3 cm.

Her goal is to get down to 112 lb and 14 percent body fat. To achieve this, she must lose 16 total pounds: 7.3 lb of fat and 8.7 lb of lean mass.

Her first follow-up is four weeks after the initial evaluation, at which time she is found to weigh 123 lb. Her body fat this time is measured as 19 percent, even though she has lost 5 lb; however, her girth measurements have decreased to upper arm: 22.8 cm, bust: 85.4 cm, waist: 65.0 cm, hips: 89.8 cm, thigh: 52.3 cm. The apparent increase in Mary Doe's percent fat is actually due to the inherent error in the method for estimating body fat, which is *plus or minus 3 percent*. We have provided this example to demonstrate that percent fat measurements should *not* be used to assess small changes in body composition.

So, although Mary Doe has lost only 5 lb and the measurement of her percent fat shows no significant change, her girth measurements show a total loss of 10.7 cm, or 4.2 inches. This indicates that Mary Doe has lost some fat and has also replaced some fat with muscle. At this point, Mary Doe and her director may wish to set up a schedule of subsequent progress evaluations for total weight and girth measurements once every four weeks, allowing another 10–12 weeks to achieve her goal of 112 lb. (We will discuss methods of weight-loss in Chapters 7 and 8.)

We're sure many readers are saying to themselves "16 weeks to lose 16 pounds! That's too long!" According to the crash-and-burn, all water-and-muscle-loss fad-diet philosophy, yes, 16 weeks is a long time. However, we are interested in permanent changes in body composition and significant losses of fat, and such changes take time.

Too Much Muscle?

It is also important to differentiate between a dancer who is overly fat and one who is overly muscular. You may ask the question "Is it possible to have too much muscle?" and find that the answer is yes. Because dancers, especially ballet dancers, must meet certain aesthetic standards, the problem of becoming too muscular is a legitimate cause for concern. Particularly because some dancers are genetically predisposed to a very mesomorphic (muscular) body type, they can often have a low percent body fat, yet still be considered "too heavy" for their company's or school's standards.

Consider the following situation; Dancer A was measured as having 11.3 percent body fat, was 63 inches tall, and weighed 99 lb. Dancer B had 12.5 percent body fat, was 64 inches tall, and weighed 133 lb. Both percent body fat levels are low; in fact, they are lower than those for most dancers. However, Dancer A is almost too thin while Dancer B is constantly admonished by her instructors to lose weight.

What should Dancer B do? This is a difficult situation to address because there has been little if any research in this particular area. One thing we do know is that often people who were once overweight and then lose weight tend to retain the extra muscle mass that was necessary to support the excess weight they once carried. However, in the case of Dancer B, there are methods she can use that may reduce her muscle bulk. She may wish to try a different technique instructor, try some training in one of the "body therapies" (i.e., Alexander, Feldenkrais, Rolfing, or Pilates), and/or the dancer may wish to take some time off dancing and focus on other activities to "reshape" her body.

It is important to appreciate that these suggestions are based solely on our experiences because there has been no research in this area. It is really a trial-and-error proposition for the dancer in trying to modify an overly muscular body. Ultimately, the dancer may have to deal with the DNA she inherited and if her mesomorphic genes win out, she would probably be best served in trying to find a company or university situation that will accept her body for the unique attributes offered by a strong, earthy quality. As prized as the sylph look is by the Balanchine school, so is the muscular look by many modern choreographers (and many dance audiences). A dancer can avoid years of self-defeating frustration by recognizing and accepting the advantages of her body type.

The Underweight Dancer

Another important consideration is the underweight dancer. In this situation, the question that should be considered is "Does this dancer have anorexia nervosa?" This is a complicated issue and we will discuss it in more detail in Chapter 9; however, not all underweight dancers have anorexia nervosa. Some may simply have difficulty maintaining a healthy dance weight. Such dancers may wish to focus on increasing their intake of complex carbohydrates and protein, and augment their dancing with appropriate weight training in an effort to improve their proportions.

In dance, the old saying "One can never be too rich or too thin" is probably more like "One can never be too turned out or too thin," but the fact is some dancers are so thin as to not only compromise their aesthetic line, but also health and performance capabilities. If weight loss continues in spite of steps to gain weight, be sure to consult a doctor to rule out the possibility of disease.

Professional Realities and Ethical Considerations

A discussion of body composition goals would not be complete without a discussion of the realities involved in professional dance. It is one thing to say a dancer needs 12–16 weeks to achieve an appropriate dance weight but it is quite another to deal with the realities of professional standards. In no way can this or any other book dictate what a school's or company's weight standards should be or how they should deal with the problem of overweight or underweight dancers. We can offer guidelines based on our current knowledge, but any dancer who reaches professional status is bound to be met by strict requirements.

Although rumors circulate of some company directors handing out amphetamines to their dancers with orders to lose weight, most directors do want to be fair to a performer who is talented and dedicated but has a weight problem. We hope that this information will serve both dancers and directors in trying to better deal with weight issues; however, because nothing can replace careful consideration and evaluation of individual situations, there is no simple problem-solving recipe.

Directors, faculty, and students in university programs should ask themselves a number of questions (some of which might also be considered by professional companies) such as: Should we have weight standards? If so, how strict should our weight standards be for performing-emphasis students?

Should we have weight standards for students going into nonperformance dance fields? What kind of policy should we have for students who don't meet weight standards? Are we familiar with appropriate referral sources for students with eating disorders? How do we strike a balance between ensuring our dancers are healthy yet meet the aesthetic standards of dance? And what *are* those aesthetic standards?

There are obviously a variety of answers to these questions; however, the important thing is that they be discussed openly among faculty and student representatives. Responsibility for setting guidelines for body weight should be shared among students, faculty, and administration, as well as the responsibility for maintaining them.

Genetic Influences on Body Composition

Research conducted by former New York City Ballet dancer Linda Hamilton (Hamilton et al., 1987; Hamilton et al., 1988) suggests that genetics play a pivotal role in how dancers respond to the demands for thinness. Hamilton compared dancers from general-audition regional companies to those who had gone through strict selection processes from early in their training, such as in company schools like School of American Ballet. She found that the highly selected dancers tended to be thinner naturally, could eat more and maintain dance weight, and had a significantly lower incidence of obesity in their families than the non-selected regional dancers.

This research underscores the pivotal role genetics play in determining a person's body composition. For those dancers interested in seeking a career with a professional ballet company, this issue should be carefully considered. Dancers who do not tend naturally towards such thinness can certainly use appropriate diet and exercise measures to help get them closer to their desired dance weight; however, sooner or later, they may have to choose between battling their inherited body traits and modifying their dance goals. For those dancers who realize they were not born with sylph-producing DNA, energy may be refocused toward dance careers that do not require an ultra-thin body, and also toward maintaining a healthy, fit body composition rather than trying to force an unhealthy skinny one.

We feel the message in this information is that an attempt should be made to provide appropriate career counseling for those dancers whose family traits do not lend themselves to strict ballet standards. Just because a dancer's body is out of the range of such requirements does not negate a career in dance. Many alternatives in performing, choreography, teaching, and dance-related careers exist that can be as fulfilling as professional ballet stage life. Perhaps most importantly, the dancer should be reassured that just because her family tree does not make her a prime candidate for a major company, it does not mean she is a failure or untalented. Positive support is essential in counseling such dancers in order to avoid a backlash of psychologically destructive behavior, and also to avoid ruining a potentially productive and successful career.

Whatever conclusions are drawn, program directors, faculty, and students should seriously consider the possible ramifications of their policies. There are simply too many dancers emotionally scarred by surprise weighings in the middle of class, humiliating remarks made by instructors in front of classmates, and other such inappropriate tactics. While nobody ever said the dance world was kind, we certainly don't need to make it more difficult than it already is. Fortunately, policies can also have a positive effect on students and/or company members, and our goal is to help provide the information necessary to design them.

Chapter IV

Overview of Nutrients

Carbohydrates, Fats, and Protein

Most dancers would like to improve their nutritional status but find it difficult to know just where they should make changes. In this chapter, carbohydrates, fats, and protein will be discussed along with recommended intakes for dancers. We will also discuss general functions of vitamins and minerals, as well as dancers' needs for iron and calcium. Understanding the function of these nutrients will be important in achieving your weight-loss or weight-maintenance goals in combination with good health. For health and weight control, it is not just how many calories you consume but also what makes up those calories that is important.

Because we cannot go into detail on every nutrient, we refer the reader to the work of Jane Brody (1983, 1981), Katch and McArdle (1983), or Krause and Mahan (1984) for further information. However, keep in mind that such nutrition texts are concerned with dietary improvements for the average person, or for someone in a disease state. As for books on nutrition for athletes, the best is *Coaches Guide to Nutrition and Weight Control* (Eisenman et al., 1989), which includes excellent information on weight control as well as some physiologic material that was beyond the scope of this book. However, while there are many similarities among dancers and athletes, dancers have certain *unique* dietary needs and problems. Therefore, we have tried to focus on those issues relevant to dancers and have limited the amount and type of information included in this book accordingly.

CARBOHYDRATES

An important distinction among carbohydrates is whether they're simple or complex. Simple carbohydrates include *monosaccharides* and *disaccharides*. Monosaccharides available from foods (glucose, fructose) are already in their simplest form and include those sugars in fruits, honey, and corn syrup. Disaccharides are two monosaccharides bonded together and are found in table sugar (sucrose) and milk (lactose).

Complex carbohydrates, *polysaccharides*, have a molecular structure that is more difficult to break down, which means it takes longer to digest and absorb them. Digestible polysaccharides are primarily made up of starch and dextrins, and are found in potatoes, wheat, corn, and other vegetables. Partially digestible polysaccharides, such as raffinose and stachyose, are found in beans and legumes.

Key points concerning carbohydrates include the following:

1. Main fuel of the central nervous system, brain, and red blood cells.
2. Protein sparing. Without carbohydrates, protein must be broken down into glucose for brain and red blood cell metabolism.
3. Needed for complete fat breakdown. In the absence of carbohydrates, fats metabolize to ketones, which are very acidic.
4. Provide fiber, which is important for the colon.
5. Bind toxins. The liver uses carbohydrates to excrete toxic substances that enter the body.
6. Provide 4 kcal of energy per gram.

Carbohydrates should constitute about 55–65 percent of total dietary intake. The average person needs about 50–100 grams of carbohydrate a day to avoid a build up of acidic ketones (ketosis). Dancers tend to eat too few carbohydrates, as we will discuss in Chapter 5.

FATS

You cannot survive on a diet completely devoid of fat (also referred to as *lipid*). Diets must contain some fat, not only for survival but for optimal health and well-being.

Key functions of fats include:

1. Main fuel in endurance aerobic state.
2. Satiety. Fat stimulates hormones that slow down gastric emptying, so food stays in stomach longer.
3. Spare protein breakdown when carbohydrate is adequate.

4. Certain fatty acids are essential in that they form part of cell walls and prostaglandins. Prostaglandins are *very important*. They affect the function of smooth muscle, and are important in recovery from injury. Essential fatty acids can be obtained from plant oils and deep sea fish oils.
5. Carry fat soluble vitamins (A, D, E, and K).
6. Form the basis of some hormones needed for adequate sexual function.
7. Supply 9 kcal of energy per gram of fat.

There are three main types of fat: (a) saturated; (b) monounsaturated; and (c) polyunsaturated. "Saturation" refers to the hydrogen content of the fat molecule. Those fatty acids that have the maximum number of hydrogen atoms associated with each carbon atom are said to be "saturated" with hydrogens, hence the name. Saturated fats tend to be solid at room temperature (such as shortening, butter, and lard). Unsaturated fats have one (mono) or more (poly) hydrogens replaced with an extra electron bond between two carbons and tend to be liquid at room temperature (corn, safflower, and other oils). Margarines made with these oils tend to be low in saturated fats.

Your diet should include both saturated and unsaturated fats. Most essential fatty acids are contained in polyunsaturated fatty acids (PUFAs), therefore, 2 to 10 percent of total dietary-adult-intake should consist of PUFAs. Intake should not exceed 10 percent because too high an intake of PUFAs causes problems related to Vitamin E. At least 10–20 percent of total dietary intake should be from fats, although a prudent diet includes up to 30 percent fat (10 percent polyunsaturated, 10 percent monounsaturated, and 10 percent saturated). Be careful if you get below a 5 percent fat intake for you may be in danger of not getting your essential fatty acids. As we shall see in Chapter 5, most dancers consume far too much fat.

PROTEIN

Protein is derived from both animal and plant sources. Unlike carbohydrates and fats, protein contains nitrogen, which enables it to form amino acids, the building blocks of living tissue. There are 22 specific amino acids, but nine of them *must* be supplied to the body through food in order to survive. These are known as *essential* amino acids. Foods that contain all nine essential amino acids are known as *complete* proteins.

Key functions of protein include:

1. Structural. Protein is the major component of muscles, tendons, ligaments, and bone matrix.
2. Fluid balance. Without protein, blood pressure forces fluid into the cells and the body becomes bloated.
3. Protein is needed to synthesize many hormones.
4. Protein is needed to form all enzymes. Enzymes are catalysts in chemical reactions.
5. Acid/base (pH) balance. Without protein the body becomes acidic.
6. Formation of antibodies.
7. Body stores of protein can be converted to glucose in starvation.
8. Protein supplies 4 kcal of energy per gram.

The average adult only needs about 0.8 grams of protein per kg body weight to stay healthy (Katch & McArdle, 1983, p. 15). To estimate your protein needs, multiply your body weight in *pounds* by 0.36. For example, a 115 lb dancer would require about 41 grams of protein a day (115 lb × 0.36 = 41.4 grams of protein).

For most people, protein should represent about 10–20 percent of the total dietary intake. Of the protein one does consume, about 20 percent needs to be "complete," that is, contain all nine essential amino acids. Complete proteins include meat, fish, and poultry; however, all nine essential amino acids can also be derived by specific combinations of nonanimal proteins. (See *Diet for a Small Planet* by Frances Moore Lappé for details on complementary proteins.) For our 115 lb dancer, 20 percent of her 41 grams of protein, or 8.2 grams, should be complete protein.

Dancers tend to consume more protein than they need. Hamilton et al. (1986) reported that female professional ballet dancers got, on average, over 177 percent of the RDA (Recommended Daily Allowance) for protein. Because many dancers also eat too few carbohydrates, some of this protein must then be converted to glucose. Too much protein is hard on the kidneys and can lead to a diet high in saturated fat if too much is from animal sources.

There continues to be controversy over how much protein a person engaged in athletic activity needs for optimal performance. Some sports-medicine nutritionists feel that protein may be lost through strenuous work and sweating, while others feel this is not significant. We have found that many female dancers have difficulty trying to lose weight with protein intakes of 10–15 percent and fat intakes below 25 percent, especially on diets under 1,200 kcal. Therefore, for the purposes of weight control, the sample diets in this book consist of approximately 20 percent protein, 20 percent fat, and 60 percent carbohydrate.

Recommended Intakes for Dancers

- **Carbohydrates: 55–65 percent of total caloric intake, should be mostly complex.**
- **Protein: 15–20 percent of total intake, 20 percent of protein intake should be essential amino acids.**
- **Fats: 15–25 percent of total intake, 2–10 percent of fat intake should be from PUFAs.**
  This is considered a low-fat diet.

Sample Intake

- **1,600 kcal/day consumed.**
- **61 percent from carbohydrates = 976 kcal per day from breads, pasta, vegetables, fruits, and cereals.**
- **19 percent from protein = 304 kcal per day from protein containing foods (which may include some breads and vegetables), and 20 percent or 61 kcal from complete proteins (chicken, fish, beef, pork, etc. or non-animal complementary proteins consumed together).**
- **20 percent from fats = 320 kcal per day from oils, salad dressings, mayonnaise, cheeses, butter, margarine, and fats in protein foods.**

Vitamins and Minerals

From Stress Formula to Flintstones, vitamin-mineral supplements are a major industry and a major part of most dancers' health care regimens. But what are vitamins and minerals?

How do they work, how do you get them in your diet, and what is the role of supplements?

Vitamins are organic compounds that are necessary for various metabolic reactions in the body and must be included in the diet. Vitamins usually function as "coenzymes"; that is, they help enzymes carry out chemical reactions. However, vitamins do *not* supply energy. Vitamins can be used over and over again so the quantities needed are very small; however, quantities in food are also small. Compositionally, there is no difference between vitamins isolated from foods and those synthesized in a laboratory although vitamins ingested from food sources are usually naturally combined with other elements that aid in absorption. Vitamins ingested separately in tablet form (whether "natural" or synthetic) may lack the necessary complements for efficient absorption. If a vitamin isn't absorbed, it cannot be used.

Minerals function as regulators. You can think of them as traffic lights of metabolism in that a proper ratio must be present in order to keep fluids, enzymes, and other compounds from getting jammed. Minerals are toxic at doses often no more than five times the RDA, much more so than vitamins, and they also tend to compete with each other for absorption, so it's important not to overdo one. It is best to get minerals from the diet for these and other reasons.

CLASSES OF VITAMINS

1. Fat soluble (A, D, E, and K): Stored in the body's fat so there is potential for toxicity, especially vitamins A and D.

2. Water soluble (B vitamins and C): Not stored in the body's fat, so little chance of toxicity. However, large doses of these vitamins can lead to problems. There's a 40–100 day supply of vitamin C in the liver so if you don't get any C for a few days, you won't get scurvy. You can store five to seven years of vitamin B_{12} in the liver.

Recommended Daily Allowance (RDA)

The RDA consists of guidelines set up by the Food and Nutrition Board of the National Research Council. The adult RDA takes into account the needs of 95 percent of the population, so the average person gets at least 45 percent over what they need if they fulfill the RDA. However, because it is impossible to tell where you fall in relationship to average, it is a good idea to follow the RDA as a general guideline to ensure adequate nutrition. Just remember, the RDA is not absolute, but it should help you determine the adequacy of your diet in general terms. RDA levels assume these nutrients are being obtained from food, not tablets, as many foods work together to increase absorption. If you're getting your RDA from supplements, you'll have to adjust your intake to account for decreased absorption.

Adequate vs. Optimal Nutrition

Consuming adequate amounts of certain nutrients is not the same as consuming those amounts which might be considered "optimal" for someone in a highly-specialized activity such as dance. Because of individual differences, it is virtually impossible in a book such as this to get too specific on what is optimal nutrition. However, in Chapter 5 we will discuss research on dancers' intakes of calories, vitamins, and minerals, which indicates that there are some common deficiencies that can and should be addressed. We will present detailed information on iron and calcium at this point because they are of particular importance to dancers.

IRON

Iron is an important part of hemoglobin, the pigment in the red blood cells that carries oxygen; and myoglobin, which carries oxygen in the muscle. Iron is also part of some enzymes and is important in the immune response. Because the oxygen-carrying capacity of your blood is directly related to how well you function, nutritional iron status is very important for dancers. If you become anemic (*anemia* is defined as a decreased oxygen-carrying capacity of the blood), you can't cure it by just eating iron-rich foods; you must take medicinal iron. A good diet can prevent but not cure anemia.

Female dancers tend to be iron-deficient, whereas male dancers tend to consume excessive amounts of iron (Cohen et al. 1985). For women, part of the problem with iron is it is not well-absorbed; you only absorb about 10 percent of what you eat. Also, some forms of dietary iron are more absorbable than others. The iron in red meats, *heme* iron, has about a 25–35 percent absorption rate. In non-red meats and plants, non-heme iron, it has only a 2–10 percent absorption rate. If the iron in your fortified cereal is iron pyrophosphate, it is not well absorbed. Ferrous sulphate or ferrous gluconate are better, which are usually in vitamins.

Eating heme iron improves the absorbability of non-heme iron when eaten together, as does vitamin C. Vitamin C can increase iron absorption up to four times, but be sure to consume iron- and vitamin C-containing foods at the same meal. This interaction is why iron RDA must be measured against vitamin C intake. Also, fructose, lactose (milk sugar), and copper increase iron absorption. The phytates and polyphenols in nuts and unleavened bread can reduce iron absorption, as can too much fiber in the diet (more than 6 grams per day of dietary fiber, not crude). Dancers who are vegetarian should be especially conscious of increasing their iron intake.

You should avoid supplementary iron when you have a bacterial or viral infection. Iron stimulates the growth of both bacteria and viruses. Supplements containing zinc should also be avoided during an infection as zinc can inhibit white cell activity.

CALCIUM

Most of the calcium in the body is inside the bone but without some calcium in the blood you would be dead. So, under normal conditions, hormones carefully regulate blood levels of calcium even if you consume no calcium in your diet. If you don't consume enough calcium, the blood gets it from your bones, which is a major factor in the development of *osteoporosis* (literally meaning "porous bone").

Key functions of calcium include:

1. Synthesis and maintenance of bones and teeth.
2. Blood clotting.
3. Muscle contraction.
4. Nerve transmission.

Every cell in the body uses calcium in controlling enzymes. Calcium is also important in the permeability of the cell membrane so that substances can cross from the bloodstream into the cell and vice versa.

Calcium in the Diet

Vitamin C, lactose, fructose, and vitamin D all increase absorption of calcium from the diet. So, eating an orange or potato with your milk, yogurt, or cottage cheese will help you absorb more calcium. Milk products are the only really good source of calcium because other sources either don't contain enough calcium or are poorly absorbed. The lactose in milk (milk sugar) and vitamin D added to milk help the absorption of calcium; however, this is a problem for people who are deficient in *lactase,* the enzyme that digests lactose. Such individuals are "lactose intolerant," and have symptoms including gas and diarrhea following the consumption of milk or milk products. However, a substance can be added to milk that digests most of the lactose, making it possible for lactase deficient individuals to consume them. (Lactaid, Inc. specializes in such products. Call toll free 800/257-8650 or write P.O. Box 111, Pleasantville, NJ 08232 for product information.)

In any case, there is no getting around the fact that without milk products you will have a very tough time getting adequate calcium by diet alone, so it is a good idea to supplement if you can't drink milk. In order to get the 800 mg RDA from supplements, you must consume about 2,000 mg in tablet form depending on the type. Sources of calcium are listed below in order of most absorbed to least absorbed.

Dietary:
1. Milk products
2. Sardines, or any fish where you get some bones
3. Legumes
4. Green vegetables (except spinach)
5. Sesame seeds

Supplements:
1. Calcium carbonate (40 percent calcium, so you get 200 mg of calcium from a 500 mg tablet—remember to adjust for this).

2. Dicalcium phosphate (31 percent calcium).
3. Calcium lactate (approximately 13 percent calcium).

Be wary of bone meal and dolomite as they may have toxic levels of lead and/or arsenic.

Osteoporosis

Osteoporosis has received a great deal of media exposure in recent years, as has the importance of calcium supplementation. Osteoporosis results in a decrease in bone density, which increases the risk of fractures. Bone density is of great importance to the dancer because it forms the crucial base of skeletal support. With a decreased bone density, the dancer is subject to fractures, scoliosis (curvature of the spine), and other skeletal problems (Benson et al., 1989; Warren et al., 1986).

The potential for this disease begins in a person's twenties and dancers are definitely in one of the highest risk categories primarily because of their light body weights, low caloric intake, and irregular menstrual periods. Women who are at risk for osteoporosis are typically light weight, caucasian (especially of Northern European descent), have a high caffeine intake, smoke, have a low intake of calcium, and menstruate less than five or six times per year. In dancers' favor is the fact that dance provides weight-bearing physical activity, which is an important defense against osteoporosis. However, poor dietary practices among dancers increases the risk for bone problems.

You are only a "bone-builder" until your mid-thirties, after that you "borrow" calcium from your peak bone mass. So, development of a high peak bone mass is very important in preventing the onset of osteoporosis. Once you have osteoporosis, there's very little you can do about it, so it is essential that dancers build and maintain their bone "bank accounts" in their teens, twenties, and early thirties.

Calcium is important in keeping-up bone density. As with any other nutrient, absorption is a pivotal factor. Two hormones regulate calcium absorption: parathyroid hormone (PTH) and calcitonin. Briefly, PTH release takes calcium out of the bone and puts it in the blood in response to low calcium levels. Calcitonin is released when there are adequate levels of calcium in the blood, and allows calcium to stay in the bone to make minerals. Because of this hormonal control, dietary intake of calcium is of critical importance.

Loss of menstruation *(amenorrhea)* is an important factor in the development of osteoporosis due to the female hormone estrogen and its influence on parathyroid hormone. Loss of menses by itself does not mean you'll get osteoporosis, but chronic poor nutrition coupled with amenorrhea for lengthy periods is a strong risk factor.

The insidious part of osteoporosis is that it is a disease that sneaks up on you in later years. A young dancer may think, "Well, I'm okay because I've never had a stress fracture," but that is no guarantee your bone structure will maintain its density as you age. In assessing their propensity for developing osteoporosis, dancers must be aware of their calcium intake, their overall nutritional status, and the frequency of their menstrual cycles. Even dancers in their twenties can suffer fractures and other injuries due to poor bone mineralization, which can threaten or end a career. We will discuss this issue further in Chapter 10, but if you find you fit the high-risk profile for osteoporosis and have been suffering from stress fractures, discuss this with a dietician, an orthopedist, and/or a physician specializing in *endocrinology* (the study of hormones).

No Magic Nutrients

Simply stated, no vitamin or mineral is a magic weight-loss formula, nor is any one nutrient more or less important than another. Dancers often get into comfortable food niches, eating the same foods day-after-day out of fear that any deviation from tried-and-true regimens will result in weight gain or a decrease in energy. Such practices limit food variety and thus compromise vitamin-mineral intake. Supplements can be helpful only if you remember that they are only supplements, not replacements. In no way can a vitamin or mineral take the place of food as an energy source.

Because of the demands for thinness, dancers tend to have specific nutritional imbalances that can negatively affect their health and performance. We will discuss these imbalances in Chapter 5, along with information on food sources of each nutrient so that you can design your diet appropriately.

Chapter V

Caloric and Nutrient Intake in Dancers

What Do Dancers Really Eat?

Everybody seems to have an opinion on what dancers *really* eat. At one dance conference the views ranged from "I just don't believe dancers really eat as little as they say they do," to "I know many dancers who live on 800 calories a day for years." So who's right?

Only in the last 10 years have scientific researchers started looking at the specific nutritional habits of adult dancers, finding (not surprisingly) inadequate diets for female dancers. (Only one study to date has also evaluated adult male dancers.) Other studies have reported on the diets of adolescent dancers, and there is even some limited information from a study of student dancers in the U.S.S.R. The results of this research for adult dancers are summarized in Table 5. 1, while the results for adolescent dancers are presented in Table 5.2.

The research studies used to compile the information on adult dancers include: Calabrese et al. (1983), Cohen et al. (1985), Hamilton et al. (1986), and White (1982). The adult dancers studied ranged in age from 15–36 years, with most about age 25. All danced with a professional company about 40 hours per week, except for the subjects of White, who danced an average of 33 hours per week.

The research studies used to compile the information on adolescent dancers include: Benson et al. (1985), Bright-See et al. (1978), and Clarkson et al. (1985). These adolescent dancers ranged in age from 12–18 years, with most about age 15. All were considered preprofessional and danced anywhere from 8–17 hours per week.

Taken as a group, these studies provide some important insights into the dynamics of diet, genetics, body composition, and dancing. While the following information does not tell us *how* to deal with the nutritional inadequacies of

Table 5.1. Summary of Caloric Intakes Among Adult Dancers

Researcher (Year)	Company (Location)	Kcal per Day (Mean)	Range
Females			
White (1982)	Ballet West (Utah)	1,282	722–2,043
Calabrese et al. (1983)	Cleveland Ballet (Ohio)	1,358	550–2,115
Cohen et al. (1985)	American Ballet Theatre (New York)	1,673	977–2,361
Hamilton et al. (1986)	Four national ballet companies (U.S.)	1,894	650–3,758
Males			
Cohen et al. (1985)	American Ballet Theatre (New York)	2,967	1,739–4,104

dancers, it does tell us *what* we're dealing with. We'll address the how later.

Dietary Intake in Adult Dancers

As you can see in Table 5.1, the female dancers of ABT and the four national ballet companies tended to have higher caloric intakes than the Cleveland Ballet or Ballet West dancers. The higher caloric intakes in the national companies might reflect the fact that these dancers come from a more highly-selected training background, which tends to favor dancers by "natural selection," that is, those who stay thin stay in. Genetic predisposition may be an important factor in this case. Another possibility is that there might be greater workloads in the rehearsals and performances of the national companies. There were no significant differences in percent body fat between the regional and national dancers.

One characteristic common to all the studies was that there was an exceptionally wide range of caloric intake among female dancers, even though body weight relative to height and percent body fat did not really vary. For example, while the mean (average) value reported by Hamilton et al. was 1,894 kcal per day, the range was from 650–3,758 kcal, even though all the dancers had similar body proportions. The authors of this study also reported that, relative to height, the dancers who weighed less actually ate more. This may be a function of some dancers being born with "thin genes" and

Table 5.2. Summary of Caloric Intakes Among Adolescent Dancers

Researcher (Year)	Location & School	Kcal per Day (Mean)	Range
Females			
Benson et al. (1985)	California Professional Schools	1,890	700–3,000 (approximate)
Clarkson et al. (1985)	Massachusetts Professional Schools	1,776	784–2,513
Bright-See et al. (1978)	Canada National Ballet School	1,867 (13–15 yrs) 1,747 (16–18 yrs)	Not reported
Kvasova (1974)	U.S.S.R. Bolshoi School	3,080	Not reported
Males			
Bright-See et al. (1978)	Canada, National Ballet School	2,382 (13–15 yrs) 2,722 (16–18 yrs)	Not reported
Kvasova (1974)	U.S.S.R. Bolshoi School	3,240	Not reported

not having to cut caloric intake as much as others to maintain their dance weight. Other possible explanations for the variation in caloric intake include differences in energy expenditure as well as differences in proportions of protein, fat, and carbohydrate in individual diets.

Certainly you could question these data by arguing that dancers wouldn't tell you what they *really* ate, but Cohen and his researchers took an extra step towards accuracy by verbally interviewing their dancer subjects in addition to asking them to keep daily food diaries. Also, Calabrese et al. had their subjects complete another diet diary a year after the initial study and found the results to be consistent with their original data.

For those dancers who reported consuming very little food, less than 800 calories a day, one might also question if periods of binging take place or if there is anorexia involved. Eating disorders are an important factor to consider, which we will discuss in more detail in Chapter 9; however, even diets of 1,300–1,900 kcal per day still leave many dancers well-below the RDA of 1,600–2,400 kcal per day, which is intended for females engaged in only light to moderate activity.

Although only one study looked at the diets of male dancers, the results indicate that they don't have anywhere near the kind of deficiencies that female dancers do. However, male dancers are also not required to be as thin, relative to average, as female dancers. Most of the males had caloric intakes well-within or above the RDA range of 2,300–3,100 kcal per day.

Dietary Intake in Adolescent Dancers

The RDA to support normal growth for girls in the age and height category of the dancers in these studies is about 2,200–2,400 kcal per day. Yet the female dancers' caloric intakes, which averaged about 1,800, were well below those requirements. The boys' intakes (2,400–2,700) were also below the RDA of from 2,800–3,200 kcal per day.

All this seems par for the course until we get to a study of Russian ballet students by Kvasova (1974). Female ballet students in the U.S.S.R., age 12–17 years, ingested an average of 3,080 kcal per day while their RDA is estimated at 3,100 kcal for 13- to 15-year-olds and 3,700 for those 16–18 years. Male ballet students ingested 3,240 kcal per day, again well-within the RDA. Obviously, this is a bit of a contrast as compared to North American dancers. Perhaps the dancers of the Bolshoi Ballet do not present the same ultra-thin look preferred in American companies; but neither are Russian dancers heavy by any standard. Unfortunately, little information in addition to these data is available that might explain the reasons for this rather striking difference in caloric intake between U.S. and U.S.S.R. dancers. We do know dancers for the Bolshoi and Kirov are highly selected from a young age, with strict attention paid to genetic endowment, and perhaps this is a major factor.

Balance of Nutrients

Another common finding among the studies for both adults and adolescents is that the dancers' diets were grossly imbalanced in terms of nutrition, especially for the women. On average, protein accounted for about 12–16 percent of these dancers' diets, carbohydrate 35–50 percent, and fat 40–55 percent. These figures show that most dancers have fat intakes that are nearly twice as high as recommended levels, with protein and carbohydrate intakes borderline or below normal levels. Even more disastrous are the individual ranges in the dancers studied by Calabrese et al.: protein intake ranged from 7–81 percent, carbohydrate from 26–82 percent, and fat from 10 to a whopping 62 percent of daily calories.

Why might this be? Do dancers really lather gobs of butter onto their morning zwieback? Actually, the high-fat intake probably comes from a misunderstanding of protein foods. Ever since the heyday of the high-protein, low-carbohydrate diets, protein has retained its halo of being a "good" food: it's okay to eat cottage cheese, a sin to eat a potato. Or so goes the myth. The problem is that a great many of these "protein" foods also contain a lot of fat, most notably cheeses, red meat, nuts, and eggs. The trend may also be based in the satiety aspects of fat (*satiety* is the feeling of being full and satisfied). Dancers, in an effort to stave off hunger pangs may gravitate towards foods they know from experience will keep them satiated through class and rehearsals.

Fortunately, the trend towards protein worship is beginning to change, but as one dancer we know put it, "I still have trouble allowing myself to eat a piece of bread." Table 5.3 compares a pseudo high-protein diet that is actually high in fat with an appropriately balanced low-fat diet. As you can see, there is a much greater variety and quantity of food ingested in the low-fat diet.

As for vitamin and mineral consumption, you might think that with such paltry caloric intakes dancers would also be depleted of essential nutrients. Not necessarily, but the roller-coaster configuration of vitamin intake is certainly eye-opening. In the study by Cohen et al., 7 of the 10 men and 11 of the 12 women took daily vitamin and mineral supplements, on which one dancer reported spending about $700 a year. This widespread use probably accounted for the fact that while dietary intake of several nutrients was low, circulating blood levels of these vitamins were usually within normal levels. The exception to this was circulating levels of ferritin (iron) for the women, which were quite low.

According to Dr. Cohen, the dependence on vitamin pills actually helped perpetuate the suboptimal dietary practices.

Table 5.3. High-Fat vs. Low-Fat Diet

Food	Calories	Fat (g)	Protein (g)	Carbohydrate (g)
HIGH FAT				
Breakfast				
1 slice Pepperidge Farm Honey Wheat Berry toast	70	1	2	13
½ Tbsp butter	55	6	0	0
Cheese omelet made with 2 eggs	160	12	12	1
1 oz Jack cheese	100	9	5	1
Lunch				
8 oz Dannon Low-Fat Blueberry Yogurt	240	3	9	44
2 Tbsp sunflower seeds	85	8	2	tr.*
3 Triscuits	70	4	1	8
Snack				
4 celery sticks	10	0	tr.	2
2 Tbsp peanut butter	190	16	9	4
Dinner				
3½ oz chicken breast, with skin, roasted	240	15	27	0
Salad: Lettuce, tomato,	20	0	0	2
1 oz Cheddar cheese,	110	9	7	1
2 Tbsp Kraft French Reduced Calorie Dressing	40	4	0	4
2 chocolate chip cookies	110	5	1	14
Totals	1500	92	75	94
Approximate Kcal		828	300	373
Percent Total Kcal		55%	20%	25%

Apparently, this dependence was due, in part, to the mistaken belief among the dancers that vitamin supplements supplied energy or wholly corrected any dietary indiscretion.

As for nutrient intake in adolescent dancers, 60 percent of the subjects of Benson et al. took vitamin-mineral supplements; however, only 7 percent took supplements that improved their nutrient status where it was needed. Many of these dancers took large doses of B vitamins, vitamin C, and vitamin A even though deficiencies were not present.

Dancers, Vitamins, and Minerals

Tables 5.4 and 5.5 list each major vitamin and mineral, its function, food sources, and the results of research on

Table 5.3. High-Fat vs. Low-Fat Diet (Continued)

Food	Calories	Fat (g)	Protein (g)	Carbohydrate (g)
LOW FAT				
Breakfast				
⅔ cup Shredded Wheat	105	0	3	23
½ cup skim milk	40	tr.	4	6
½ grapefruit	40	0	0	10
Snack				
1 cup cubed cantaloupe	60	0	0	15
1 small bran muffin	100	4	1	15
½ cup skim milk	40	tr.	4	6
Lunch				
Sandwich made with 1½ oz lean roast beef,	80	4	10	0
2 slices Roman Meal bread,	140	2	6	25
½ Tbsp Hellman's "Light" mayonnaise,	25	2	0	1
Lettuce, tomato	10	0	0	2
1 cup steamed broccoli	50	0	4	8
6 oz pineapple juice	100	0	tr.	25
Snack				
¼ cup wheat germ mixed with	110	3	8	13
8 oz Kraft Light n' Lively Strawberry Yogurt	160	2	7	29
Dinner				
Salad made with spinach, mushrooms, sprouts, tomato	20	0	tr.	5
½ Tbsp olive oil,	60	7	0	0
vinegar, or lemon juice	tr.	0	0	tr.
3½ oz broiled turkey breast, skinless	110	3	21	0
1 cup spaghetti squash	30	0	2	5
½ Tbsp margarine	55	6	0	0
1 baked medium potato	95	tr.	3	21
1 Strawberry Frozfruit bar	70	0	tr.	16
Totals	1500	33	78	225
Approximate Kcal		297	312	900
Percent Total Kcal		19%	21%	60%

*tr. = trace.

Table 5.4. Vitamins: Functions, Sources, & Dancers' Intakes

Function	Sources	Dancers' Intakes	Comments
Fat Soluble Vitamins			
VITAMIN A Needed for light reaction in the eyes; helps protect gut, eyes, and skin; helps maintain immune system; and is important in growth and development of long bones.	Liver, carrots, sweet potatoes, spinach, apricots, winter squash, cantaloupe, broccoli, crab, peaches.	*Adequate.* Generally, adult and adolescent dancers appear to get adequate amounts of vitamin A from their diets. Although Bright-See et al. (1978) found a number of their adolescent ballet dancers inadequate in vitamin A intake, more recent studies show the opposite trend with some dancers well into overdose levels.	Vitamin A is toxic at 200 times the RDA for a single dose, but it is toxic at only 10 times the RDA if ingested chronically. That is, someone taking 18,500 to 60,000 IU/day in synthetic water-soluble form over a period of several months can become toxic.
VITAMIN D Aids in the formation and maintenance of bones and teeth, and assists in the absorption of calcium.	Vitamin D can be acquired either by ingesting vitamin D-containing foods (an inefficient source) or by exposure to sunlight (an efficient source). To get enough vitamin D, you need about 15 minutes a day of sunlight. Most milk is fortified with Vitamin D.	*Inadequate.* Vitamin D was found to be deficient both dietarily and after supplementation in the majority of dancers studied by Calabrese et al. Cohen et al. also found dancers' diets to be deficient in vitamin D, but this was corrected by supplements taken by their dancers. A major difference between the subjects in these two	

Vitamin	Function	Food Sources	Studies	Toxicity
(Vitamin D, continued)			studies is that the Calabrese et al. group took one of three general supplements whereas the Cohen et al. group consumed "extraordinary amounts" of vitamin pills. If increasing exposure to sunlight is not possible, dancers should consider adjusting their diets and/or specifically (but carefully) supplementing vitamin D.	There is a significant possibility of vitamin D overdose with fish oils or vitamin supplements. Four to ten times the RDA (800 to 2,000 IU) is toxic if ingested in the diet. Sunlight, however, cannot be toxic for vitamin D because the liver inactivates any excess.
VITAMIN E	Vitamin E's major function is as an antioxidant; that is, it prevents oxygen, water, and other oxidizing agents from destroying cell membranes and prevents rancidity in foods.	Corn oil, cottonseed oil, soy oil, margarines, almonds, soy beans, wheat germ.	*Possibly Inadequate.* Only Benson et al. have reported on vitamin E intake in dancers (adolescents) and they felt intake was inadequate in 38 percent of their subjects.	Too much E can inhibit prostaglandin synthesis (important factor in healing) and blood platelet formation. Doses over 600 IU/day have caused significant reduction in thyroid hormone and elevation of serum triglyceride (part of the fat molecule) levels in females.
VITAMIN K	You can forget about K because your gut makes it. You only need to worry about vitamin K if you're an infant or there's something wrong with your intestines.	Broccoli, cabbage, lettuce, turnip greens.		

Table 5.4. Vitamins: Functions, Sources, & Dancers' Intakes (Continued)

Function	Sources	Dancers' Intakes	Comments
WATER SOLUBLE VITAMINS. These vitamins are not normally stored in the body and a daily supply is desirable to avoid depletion.			
THIAMIN (VITAMIN B_1)			
Needed for metabolism of carbohydrates, fats, and proteins, but especially carbohydrate metabolism in the brain.	Lean pork, wheat germ, liver, lean meats, poultry, egg yolk, peanuts, whole grains.	*Adequate.* According to the research, dancers receive plentiful amounts of thiamine from diet alone.	
RIBOFLAVIN (VITAMIN B_2)			
Essential for energy metabolism, growth, corticosteroids, red blood cells, formation of glucose from other substrates (like protein), and thyroid function.	Milk, cottage cheese, lean meats, eggs, green leafy vegetables.	*Adequate.* As with thiamine, dancers in general seem to fare well in terms of riboflavin from diet alone.	
NIACIN			
Helps form central components of energy metabolism.	Lean meats, poultry, fish, peanuts and peanut butter, brewer's yeast.	*Adequate with Supplementation.* Cohen et al. observed that dancers were slightly deficient in their intake of niacin dietarily but improved their status to at least 75 percent of the RDA with supplementation. A general vitamin supplement should be adequate.	

VITAMIN B_6

Function	Food Sources	Research Findings	Recommendations
Needed to build amino acids. The reason we only need to eat only 9 out of the 22 known amino acids is because B_6 helps us build the other 13. Also important in the synthesis of hemoglobin (oxygen carrying part of red blood cells), and maintenance of the nervous and immune systems.	Yeast (dry active), sunflower seeds, wheat germ, beef liver, soybeans, walnuts, salmon, light meat chicken, brown rice, bananas.	*Inadequate.* Calabrese et al. found all their dancers deficient dietarily and almost two-thirds deficient even after supplementation. Benson et al. also found their adolescent dancers deficient in B_6. However, while Cohen et al. found inadequate intake from diet alone, their group's status was improved to at least 75 percent of the RDA after supplementation.	Proper B_6 dietary adjustments and supplementation are recommended, but care should be taken because overdoses (100 mg) of B_6 can cause problems such as sleepiness.

FOLIC ACID (ALSO REFERRED TO AS FOLATE OR FOLACIN)

Function	Food Sources	Research Findings	Recommendations
Cell division, formation and maturation of red and white blood cells in the bone marrow, synthesis of genetic material.	Wheat germ, brewer's yeast, wheat bran, egg yolk, liver, spinach, romaine lettuce, orange juice, cabbage, almonds, whole wheat bread, broccoli, bananas.	*Very Inadequate.* One area in which all investigators are in agreement is that dancers are deficient in folic acid both dietarily and after supplementation. It is important to get more folic acid into your diet because it is more absorbable from foods than from supplements. As for supplements, try to find one that has 600–800 µg of folic acid.	This vitamin is very commonly deficient in the U.S. diet, probably because folic acid is not very absorbable in some foods. In tablet form, it is only about 50 percent absorbable.

Table 5.4. Vitamins: Functions, Sources, & Dancers' Intakes (Continued)

Function	Sources	Dancers' Intakes	Comments
VITAMIN B$_{12}$			
Formation of red blood cells, building of genetic material, functioning of nervous system. B$_{12}$ is also needed for proper folic acid metabolism, so if you lack B$_{12}$, you get all the problems associated with a folic acid deficiency as well. A B$_{12}$ deficiency is more serious because it can result in nerve degeneration.	Beef liver, clams, oysters, meat, fish, eggs, chicken.	*Inadequate without Supplementation.* From diet alone, Cohen et al. found most of their dancers to be deficient in B$_{12}$; however, this was corrected by the dancers' supplementation (remember, this group consumed extreme amounts of vitamins). Be sure to check the label of your supplement since Calabrese et al. found 61 percent of their dancers deficient even after supplementation.	B$_{12}$ is only in animal foods, so vegetarians must supplement their diets.
PANTOTHENIC ACID			
Important in aerobic metabolism, as well as other metabolic functions.	Liverwurst, Cheerios, wheat germ, chicken, tomato sauce, sweet potatoes, white potatoes, oatmeal.	*Inadequate without Supplementation:* Calabrese et al. found 79 percent of their dancers deficient even after supplementation, although Cohen et al. found their dancers had adequate intakes with supplementation.	

VITAMIN C

Helps maintain connective tissue, aids in iron absorption, helps maintain immune system and cell structure, and is needed for proper folic acid metabolism.	Citrus fruits, kiwis, tomatoes, strawberries, cantaloupe, green peppers, potatoes (baked with skin), broccoli.	*Adequate.* Vitamin C is probably the one nutrient dancers get in abundance, both dietarily and with supplements. If anything, some dancers may be at risk for overconsumption of C at the expense of other nutrients.	High doses of vitamin C can be detrimental to health. More than 1,000–2,000 mg (or 1–2 grams) of vitamin C a day can cause: 1. Overabsorption of iron, which can cause liver problems. 2. Withdrawal scurvy. The body gets so used to large doses of C it responds by not conserving it well. If you've been taking high doses of C, slowly cut down to normal so your body can readjust. 3. Excess C is excreted in the urine as reductones. In the past, these have been claimed to be health promoting and although no one is really sure, they are not as benign as once thought.

It is recommended that C intake be no higher than 250 mg/day under any circumstances. As for vitamin C and the common cold, according to Krause and Mahan (1984, p. 134), "Large doses of vitamin C may have small effects on the severity and duration of the symptoms of a cold and the effect seems to be greater in females, especially young females."

BIOTIN

Essential for the activity of many enzymes, as well as metabolism of fatty acids.	Liver, mushrooms, peanuts, yeast, milk, meat, egg yolk, most vegetables, bananas, grapefruit, tomato, watermelon, strawberries.	*Inadequate.* Calabrese et al. and Cohen et al. found low biotin intake in dancers both dietarily and after supplementation. Although the exact levels needed are difficult to establish, be sure your vitamin supplement includes the recommended levels of biotin and adjust your diet accordingly.

Table 5.5. Minerals: Functions, Sources, and Dancers' Intakes

Function	Sources	Dancers' Intakes	Comments
IRON			
Formation of hemoglobin in blood and myoglobin in muscles, which supply oxygen to cells.	Liver, red meats, egg yolk, green leafy vegetables, dried fruits, blackstrap molasses, potatoes.	*Inadequate (see Chapter 4 for details).* Both dietarily and after supplementation, female dancers are very deficient in iron.	
CALCIUM			
Building and maintenance of bone and teeth strength, muscle contraction, cell membranes, blood clotting.	Milk and milk products, sardines, dark green leafy vegetables.	*Inadequate (see Chapter 4 for details).* Although Cohen et al. found their subjects had adequate intakes of calcium with supplementation, intake from diet alone was inadequate in all studies.	
PHOSPHORUS			
Phosphorus constitutes about 80 percent of the inorganic part of bones and teeth. Phosphorus is also important in the body's acid-base (pH) regulation.	Cheese, eggs, milk, meat, fish, whole grains.	*Usually Adequate.* Cohen et al. found their adult dancers' diets contained plenty of phosphorus. However, Benson et al. found inadequate phosphorus intakes in 17 percent of their adolescent dancers. One reason might be the higher RDA for adolescents.	
MAGNESIUM			
About 50 percent of the body's magnesium is in bone, with almost all the remaining 50 percent inside body cells. Magnesium functions as an activator of many enzymes.	Whole grain cereals, nuts, meat, milk, dark green vegetables.	*Inadequate.* Only Benson et al. have looked at dancers' (adolescent) magnesium intakes but they did find a marked inadequacy. Supplementing magnesium may be warranted for the adult dancer as well.	

Table 5.5. Minerals: Functions, Sources, and Dancers' Intakes *(Continued)*

Function	Sources	Dancers' Intakes	Comments
ZINC			
Zinc is important in enzyme function and it plays a crucial role in the synthesis of proteins.	Milk, liver, shellfish, herring, wheat bran.	*Inadequate.* Again, only Benson et al. recorded zinc intakes but they found it to be one of the most profoundly deficient elements in their dancers' diets. Supplementation is recommended.	Zinc has recently received a great deal of attention regarding its importance if you are "stressed," exercising heavily, want to avoid a cold, or recover more quickly from infection. However, be aware that all these supposed "benefits". of zinc are merely theories; no one really knows if or how it works in these situations.
SODIUM			
Sodium is important in the regulation of body fluid, acid-base balance, and is an important part of extracellular fluid.	Table salt, seafood.	*No data.* Dancers should be sure their sodium intake is adequate if they are rehearsing, performing, and therefore, sweating a great deal.	Sodium is often featured in the media as the major culprit in high blood pressure, although cross-cultural studies show the link between salt and blood pressure to be, at most, a weak one. American processed foods are high in sodium (4 oz of condensed *Campbell's Homestyle Chicken Noodle* soup contains 910 mg of sodium) as are many "fast food" offerings.

Table 5.5. Minerals: Functions, Sources, and Dancers' Intakes *(Continued)*

Function	Sources	Dancers' Intakes	Comments
POTASSIUM			
Potassium functions in regulating acid-base balance, fluid balance, and cell membrane transfer, and is necessary for carbohydrate and protein metabolism. Along with sodium and chlorine, it makes up what are called *electrolytes,* which are important in maintaining normal muscle function.	Fruits, milk, meat, cereals, vegetables, legumes.	*Adequate with Exceptions.* Benson et al. found their adolescent dancers had adequate intakes of both sodium and potassium. However, these levels can drop to dangerously low levels during fasting or illness (due to vomiting). Be sure to replenish your sodium and potassium levels if you are in either of these situations.	

OTHER MINERALS

Iodine, with an RDA of 150 μg, is important to thyroid function and is found in iodized table salt, seafood, water, and many vegetables. Other essential minerals and their Adequate Daily Allowances include:

Manganese, 2.5–5.0 mg
Fluoride, 1.5–4.0 mg

Molybdenum, 0.15–0.5 mg
Cobalt, a constituent of vitamin B_{12}, 3.0 μg of B_{12}

Selenium, 0.05–0.2 mg
Chromium, 0.05–0.2 mg

Other essential trace elements with no known recommended levels include: Arsenic, tin, nickel, vanadium, and silicon.

Table 5.6. RDAs and Summary of Vitamin Intakes Among Dancers

Vitamin	RDA	Dancers' Intake
A	800 RE* or 4,000 IU† (women) 1,000 RE or 5,000 IU (men)	Adequate
D	400 IU or 10 μg** (adolescents) 200 IU or 5 μg (adults)	Adequate Inadequate
E	10–20 IU or 8–10 mg alpha–TE (Depends on PUFA intake)	Possibly Inadequate
B₁ (Thiamine)	0.5 mg/1,000 kcal or 1.0–1.5 mg	Adequate
B₂ (Riboflavin)	0.6 mg/1,000 kcal or 1.2–1.7 mg	Adequate
Niacin	13–19 mg	Adequate
B₆	2.0–2.2 mg	Inadequate
Folic Acid	400 μg	Inadequate
B₁₂	3.0 μg	Inadequate
Pantothenic Acid††	4–7 mg	Inadequate
C	60 mg	Adequate
Biotin††	100–300 μg	Inadequate

Dancers' Intake based on dietary intake with general multivitamin supplement.
*RE = Retinol Equivalents
†IU = International Units
**μg = micrograms
††No RDA, adequate daily amount.

Table 5.7. RDAs and Summary of Mineral Intakes Among Dancers

Mineral	RDA	Dancers' Intake
Iron	18 mg–women 10 mg–men	Inadequate Adequate
Calcium	800 mg, but 1,000 mg recommended for dancers	Inadequate
Phosphorus	800 mg (adult) 1,200 mg (age 11–18)	Adequate Inadequate
Magnesium	300–350 mg	Inadequate
Zinc	15 mg	Inadequate
Sodium††	1,100–3,300 mg	Adequate
Potassium††	1,875–5,625 mg	Adequate

Dancers' Intake based on dietary intake with general multivitamin-mineral supplement.
††No RDA, adequate daily amount.

dancers' intakes. Warnings regarding toxicity from overdose are provided where appropriate. We have already discussed two nutrients, iron and calcium, in Chapter 4. The RDAs for vitamins and minerals relative to dancers' intakes are presented in Tables 5.6 and 5.7.

The Need for Quality Nutrition

Because dance does not burn significant numbers of calories, many female dancers must cut their caloric intake to maintain their dancing weight. Therefore, if caloric intake must be low, then the quality of that intake should indeed be high. This aspect is especially important for the young dancer for whom development of bone mass is critical. In any case, there is a great need for sound, relevant, nutritional counseling that does not dismiss dancers' professional body composition standards as frivolous.

So, our purpose in relating the information from these studies is so the individual dancer can generate a clear idea of how she or he compares to other dancers, both in terms of nutritional consumption and body composition. Broadening the variety of foods ingested, with attention paid to high-quality substances, is perhaps the simplest, most effective way of improving your nutritional status. However, because this can be especially difficult to the dancer with a low caloric intake, target your food choices for those areas where dancers tend to be deficient (or where you find yourself deficient), and choose an appropriate vitamin-mineral supplement if needed.

Chapter VI

Understanding the Exercise Demands of Dance

Why Dancing Does Not Promote Weight Loss

How many times have we all heard it: "How can you have trouble losing weight with all that *dancing* you do?" As we said in Chapter 2, dancing gives the appearance of being the kind of exercise that would burn up loads of calories, but unfortunately this is not the case. Because dance is primarily *anaerobic*—that is, short-duration, high-intensity—it simply does not promote high energy consumption or fat burning.

So does this mean dancers are wimps? Certainly not, but what about dancers being the most "physically fit" of all athletes? Although it's true that dancers have been found to be second only to professional football players in terms of *overall* demands on their bodies (Nicholas, 1975), we must carefully define what we mean by "physically fit."

When we look at the total demands of dance, including strength, flexibility, cardiovascular endurance, fine-motor coordination, and timing, professional dance rates as one of the most physically demanding activities you can do. However, while dancers on average possess extraordinary flexibility, coordination, timing, and strength in certain muscle groups, their cardiovascular endurance capabilities are more along the lines of ordinary.

Cardiovascular fitness is measured by the maximal amount of oxygen absorbed while performing a physically demanding activity. In technical terms, this is referred to as "maximal oxygen uptake" and is abbreviated $\dot{V}O_{2\,max}$. $\dot{V}O_{2\,max}$ is commonly referred to as maximal aerobic power.

Generally speaking, the higher a person's $\dot{V}O_{2\,max}$, the greater the cardiovascular fitness. By measuring $\dot{V}O_{2\,max}$ in the general population as well as in various types of athletes, we can get a good idea of the physical demands of a particular sport or activity. All this ties into understanding the energy requirements of dance class, rehearsal, and performance. Measurements of $\dot{V}O_{2\,max}$ taken during these activities tell us a great deal about how dancers expend energy, and also how they don't.

Energy Requirements of Dance

Dr. Jerald Cohen, a cardiologist with an avid interest in dancers, has conducted a number of studies on the cardiovascular characteristics of dancers. By strapping a portable, open-circuit spirometry system onto dancers, Dr. Cohen was able to measure just how much oxygen is consumed during class (Cohen et al., 1982c). Heart rates were also measured by means of radio telemetry, which involved small wireless heart rate monitors strapped to the dancers' chests.

The subjects were 15 male and female dancers from American Ballet Theatre. Their typical class consisted of 28 minutes of barre work and 32 minutes of center floor work. Based on the oxygen consumption and heart rate measurements, Dr. Cohen found that the average net caloric expenditure for women during the one-hour class was just 200 kcal for women and 300 kcal for men.

Dr. Cohen also measured heart rates during actual performances of *Swan Lake*, *Giselle*, *Etudes*, and *La Bayadere* (Cohen et al., 1982b). In order to establish how hard someone is working, heart rates are compared to a maximum, which is determined according to age. (The general equation is 220 − age in years = "age-predicted maximum heart rate.") Heart rate during the activity is then expressed as a percent of maximum. For example, a 21-year-old would have an age-predicted maximum heart rate of 199 beats per minute (bpm) whereas a 31-year-old would have an age-predicted max of 189 bpm. If during a certain activity, the 21-year-old's heart rate reached 165 bpm, that person would be working at 83 percent of age-predicted max. At 165 bpm, the 31-year-old would be working at 87 percent of age-predicted max. There are more precise equations for making this determination, which take into account resting heart rate, but this is the general idea.

Without going into the details of how heart rate rose in response to each piece of choreography, Dr. Cohen's study showed the following trends:

1. **Actual time spent dancing was anywhere from 14–30 percent of total performance time, with the longest single period of non-stop dancing being 7 minutes.**
2. **Average heart rate during the dancing periods ranged from 70–88 percent of age-predicted max, but peak heart rate often reached 95–100 percent of max.**
3. **The overall performance demands tended to fall into the category of interval work; that is, 2 to 3 minutes of intense activity followed by 2 to 3 minutes of rest (both onstage and off).**

From this and other studies, researchers have classified dance as a short-duration, high-intensity activity. This is in contrast to endurance activity where heart rate will average 60–70 percent of age-predicted max over a period of 30 minutes or more of continuous exercise.

These findings in no way mean dancers are not in good cardiovascular condition. Interval work is actually excellent conditioning for the heart. However, it does mean that, in general, dance is not an activity that promotes fat-utilization or that burns up large numbers of calories.

Aerobic Fitness

As previously mentioned, the overall cardiovascular or aerobic fitness of an individual is determined by measuring their $\dot{V}O_{2\,max}$. There are several methods for doing this, but the most often used is the treadmill "stress test." You may have read about such tests in articles about rehabilitation for victims of heart attacks, but stress tests are also used to determine the fitness levels of people who participate in various kinds of activity. The basic idea is to strap a mask onto the person's face to collect all the exhaled air (which is then analyzed for its oxygen and carbon dioxide content), put them on a motorized treadmill, and have them walk or run to exhaustion.

By comparing the results of these treadmill tests, we can get an idea of where dancers rank on the cardiovascular fitness spectrum. Figure 6.1 shows a graphic comparison of a number of $\dot{V}O_{2\,max}$ values from various studies of dancers and some general classifications of female athletes. ($\dot{V}O_{2\,max}$ can be adjusted for body weight and is measured in units of milliliters of oxygen per kilogram of body weight per minute

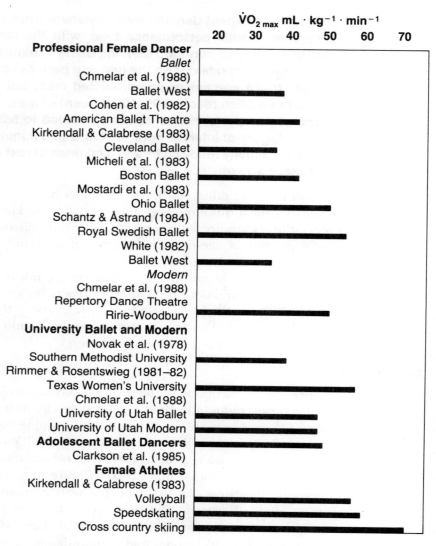

Figure 6.1. Comparison of $\dot{V}O_{2max}$ Values in Female Dancers and Athletes

of exercise, which is notated $mL \cdot kg^{-1} \cdot min^{-1}$.) Although there is a range of values among dancers depending on the group studied and the testing protocol used, most female dancers who train regularly have a $\dot{V}O_{2\,max}$ between 40 and 45 $mL \cdot kg^{-1} \cdot min^{-1}$. Male dancers are not included in the graph, but their $\dot{V}O_{2\,max}$ values tend to be in the high-40s to low-50s. As compared to athletes such as cross-country skiers, who have average $\dot{V}O_{2\,max}$ values in the 70s and 80s, dancers would be classified as nonendurance. In general, in order to be classified in an endurance category, $\dot{V}O_{2\,max}$ for females needs to be at least 50 ml $\cdot$ kg^{-1} $\cdot$ min^{-1}.

In our study comparing levels and styles of dancers, we found that the professional ballet dancers from our area had lower $\dot{V}O_{2\,max}$ values than university ballet and modern dancers or professional modern dancers. This led to some interesting speculation as to just what might account for this difference in aerobic power.

Because aerobic power is dependent on variables such as how much you train, the kind of training, genetic predilection, age, and sex, a higher $\dot{V}O_{2\,max}$ average in one group over another would lead one to examine possible differences in these variables, especially training. For example, did the professional ballet dancers we studied train less intensively than either of the university groups or the professional modern dancers? Well, the lower aerobic power capabilities would lead one to think so, but it is more important to examine the possible reasons for this. Some of the questions we asked included:

- Were there more injuries among the professional ballet dancers? Yes; in fact, 44 percent of them had experienced a major injury in the year prior to the study vs. only 22 percent or less of the other dancers.
- Were there more dancers in the professional ballet company and perhaps less time spent dancing by some of them because of competition? "Yes" to the first part of the question and "possibly" to the second part. There were about 25 female dancers in the professional ballet company, four in each of the two professional modern companies, and about 10 each in the university ballet and modern student performing groups studied. With fewer dancers to fill all roles in the repertory, the dancers from the professional modern and university companies might have done more dancing.
- Did the director of the professional ballet dancers focus more attention on principals and soloists than corps dancers, leading to more "on the sidelines" time for corps members? This is hard to say, but we do know that different

directors have distinct styles in how they conduct rehearsals. Some favor a system where the principals and soloists are rehearsed the most, whereas others spend more time with the corps, and vice versa.

- Were there differences in extra training activities among the groups? Yes; 89 percent of the professional modern dancers, who had the highest $\dot{V}O_{2\,max}$, reported engaging in some form of aerobic training in addition to their dancing, whereas only 33 percent of the professional ballet group did so. Of the university groups, 50 percent of the ballet and 60 percent of the modern dancers practiced some form of aerobic training.
- Did the demands of choreography differ greatly among the groups? In our study, we didn't find that stylistic differences were much of a factor; however, for other groups, it might be. As previously mentioned, some contemporary choreographers work in a type of endurance style. Dancers of such choreography might be expected to have higher aerobic fitness levels than those who perform more traditional choreography.

So, variations in training among different groups of dancers can significantly affect aerobic fitness, with some or all of the reasons listed above probably responsible for these variations. However, in terms of aerobic fitness, most dancers fall into the category of "good" or "excellent" as compared to other non-athletic groups, but they fall into the "nonendurance" category as compared to athletes.

Anaerobic Fitness

In Chapter 2, we discussed the differences between aerobic and anaerobic metabolism, as well as aerobic and anaerobic exercise. We also discussed that dance is an anaerobic activity. The question then is "Are dancers anaerobically fit?" To answer this question we must first define anaerobic fitness and then describe the ways it can be measured.

First, a review of the basics of anaerobic energy production is in order. Remember that anaerobic metabolism is called upon in situations of high energy demand and results in the formation of lactic acid (also referred to as lactate). The harder you work, the more lactic acid is formed; and the more lactic acid you can form, the more anaerobically fit you are. So, the amount of lactic acid present in the blood at the completion of a maximal short-term exercise bout is a good indication of anaerobic fitness.

We'd like to take this opportunity to say a few kind words about lactic acid. Lactic acid has been held responsible for such infirmities as delayed muscle soreness, bloating, over-developed muscles, and lack of flexibility. The fact is, lactic acid is not responsible for any of these. Actually, if you didn't have lactic acid, you couldn't dance. The reason is that in order to continue energy production, a substance called NADH (nicotinamide adenine dinucleotide) must be recycled in its positive form: NAD +. The formation of lactic acid allows this NAD + to be recycled and energy production to continue. The concentration of lactic acid in the muscle cell must be kept low, and this is done by pumping lactic acid into the blood. When the concentration of lactic acid in the blood gets too high, the lactic acid in the cell piles up and the recycling of NAD + cannot continue. Without a supply of NAD +, energy production grinds to a halt.

The build-up of lactic acid in the blood indirectly contributes to fatigue during an intense work bout, but as soon as you rest the lactic acid is sent quickly on its way *out* of the body (via the heart and lungs), or it is converted to glucose (by skeletal muscle and the liver). So the idea of lactic acid hanging around in your muscles and making you sore is not correct. Although we won't get into the details here, muscle soreness that sets in a day or two after an intense work-out is actually due primarily to microtears in the muscle fibers resulting from sudden overwork. In effect, millions of microscopic muscle pulls occur, which lead to inflammation, stiffness, and soreness.

Through training, the body can increase its tolerance for greater amounts of lactic acid in the blood. The more highly trained a person is anaerobically, the more lactic acid can build up in the blood, which means you can do more anaerobic work before fatigue sets in. In other words, dancers who can tolerate high blood levels of lactic acid can execute demanding variations with less fatigue. So, the much maligned lactic acid molecule is actually one of a dancer's staunchest allies.

In order to determine anaerobic fitness, the amount of lactic acid in the blood is measured after a short, maximal work-out. This is done by taking a blood sample before and after the work-out, and then analyzing it for its lactic acid concentration. The higher the level, the greater the ability to do anaerobic work.

The relative demands of different activities can also be determined by measuring blood lactic acid, much as Dr. Cohen did with measuring heart rates and oxygen consumption during class. Drs. Schantz and Åstrand measured blood levels of lactic acid in female dancers of the Royal Swedish Ballet accumulated during class and rehearsal, as well as during a maximal-effort treadmill test.

During barre and center floor warm-up, the dancers' lactic acid levels rose to only 3.0 millimoles per liter of blood (mmol/L). (Don't worry about what a millimole is.) This is fairly low, as resting blood lactic acid levels are about 1.0–2.0 mmol/L. During rehearsal, while sections of choreography were being run, the dancers averaged 8.2 mmol/L, which is a substantial increase. After the maximal treadmill run, the dancers lactic acid averaged 11.2 mmol/L, which is high for females and indicates a good to excellent level of anaerobic fitness.

Figure 6.2 compares the blood lactic acid levels of various dance groups and athletes. These comparisons are a little difficult to make because different testing protocols can significantly affect results. However, it suffices to say that it appears most dancers who train regularly have a high level of anaerobic fitness, although we did find the professional ballet dancers in our study to have lower lactic acid levels than the university ballet or modern dance groups.

So, while dancers may not be "super-athletes" in terms of their aerobic fitness, they can have excellent levels of anaerobic fitness. A high level of anaerobic fitness is extremely important for the dancer to be able to execute allegro variations, jumping sequences, and other high-intensity sections of choreography. Unfortunately, being anaerobically fit does not promote low levels of body fat in the same way aerobic fitness does.

With aerobic fitness, the higher the $\dot{V}O_{2\,max}$ of an individual, the lower the percent body fat. Several studies of

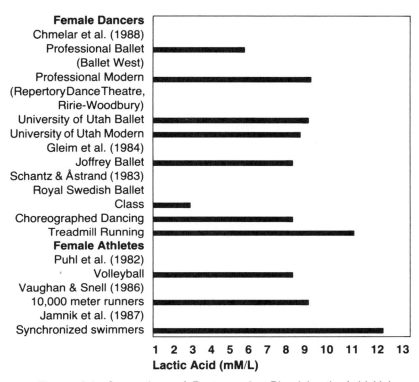

Figure 6.2. Comparison of Post-exercise Blood Lactic Acid Values Among Female Dancers and Athletes

dancers have supported this, showing that those dancers who have greater aerobic power also have lower levels of body fat. The same relationship does not hold true for anaerobic fitness, however.

Although it is also important for dancers to be anaerobically fit, it is primarily by increasing your aerobic fitness that you become a better fat burner. With increased aerobic fitness, metabolic rate increases, fat burning is increased during endurance exercise, and body fat levels decrease. In order to increase aerobic fitness and enhance fat loss, endurance activities should be emphasized.

As we introduced in Chapter 2 and will discuss further in Chapter 8, all aerobic exercise is not equal when it comes to promoting fat loss. But before we go into the specifics of the type of exercise that *will* increase your fat losses, we will next discuss the specifics of diet.

Chapter VII

Dietary Guidelines to Promote Fat Loss

At this point, we could lie and say that if you'll just follow everything this book says you'll be guaranteed to achieve your ideal dance body in a few short weeks and keep it that way. Unfortunately, no one can honestly guarantee such results; however, we can provide guidelines specifically designed for dancers based on the most up-to-date research available that will help you make the best possible choices concerning your weight control efforts.

It should be clear by now that no single food source can be eliminated in order to magically melt away fat. However, a reduced-calorie diet that is high in nutrients and low in fat combined with consistent, long-duration aerobic exercise has proven to be *the* most successful regimen for weight loss. The problem is, how do you ensure that your diet is nutritionally sound while cutting calories?

As we have discussed previously, carbohydrate, protein, and fat need to be well-balanced for optimal losses of body fat. However, each of these groupings can be further categorized according to fruit, vegetables, and bread (carbohydrate); milk, meat, poultry, and fish (protein); and plant oils, cheese, and nuts (fat). Incorporating proper ratios into each of these subgroups is how you can ensure that your diet provides you with needed vitamins and minerals while you're losing fat.

The Exchange System

One of the most effective guides to diet planning is known as the Exchange System. This meal planning approach groups food into six basic categories:

1. **STARCH/BREAD**
2. **MEAT (a) LEAN, (b) MEDIUM-FAT, (c) HIGH-FAT**
3. **VEGETABLE**
4. **FRUIT**
5. **MILK (a) SKIM, (b) LOW-FAT, (c) WHOLE**
6. **FAT**

Each major food grouping corresponds to approximate caloric, carbohydrate, protein, and fat contents, which are listed in Table 7.1 . A complete list of exchange foods for each group is provided in Appendix A.

There is no set rule for caloric intake using the Exchange System; rather, you decide on the caloric intake, and then match up the correct number of exchanges. Table 7.2 provides diet plans based on balanced exchanges corresponding to specific caloric intakes. The exchange plans we list comprise low-fat diets, which are intended to promote weight loss or maintain a below-normal weight. Therefore, only lean meat and skim milk products are used in these plans. Complete exchange menus for caloric intakes from 1,000–2,000 kcal per day are listed in Appendix D.

Now, some of you may laugh at the idea of trying to lose weight on a diet of 1,000 kcal when you currently maintain your weight on 800. But remember, these diets are quite low in fat, which makes a big difference in the body's metabolism. If you already have a caloric intake below 1,000 kcal and have not been successful at losing weight, try the 1,000 kcal *low-fat* diet we recommend and increase your exercise levels according to the guidelines in Chapter 8. In general, we don't recommend diets under 1,000 kcal because of the associated problems with deficient nutrient status, but if you

Table 7.1. Breakdown of Exchanges by Caloric, Carbohydrate, Protein, and Fat Content*

Exchange Group	Kcal (approx)	Carbohy-drate (g)	Protein (g)	Fat (g)
STARCH	80	15	3	TR
MEAT				
LEAN	55	0	7	3
MEDIUM-FAT	75	0	7	5
HIGH-FAT	100	0	7	8
VEGETABLE	25	5	2	0
FRUIT	60	15	0	0
MILK				
SKIM	90	12	8	TR
LOW-FAT	120	12	8	5
WHOLE	150	12	8	8
FAT	45	0	0	5

*Values are approximate.

Table 7.2. Balanced Low-fat Daily Caloric Intakes on the Exchange Plan*

Total (kcal)	STARCH (Exch)	LEAN MEAT† (Exch)	VEGETABLE (Exch)	FRUIT (Exch)	SKIM MILK† (Exch)	FAT (Exch)
1,000	3.5	2.5	5	2.5	2	3
1,200	4.5	3	5	3	2.5	3.5
1,350	5	3.5	5	3	2.5	4
1,500	6	4	5	4	3	4
1,650	7	4.5	5	4	3	4.5
1,800	7.5	5	5	5	3	5
2,000	9	5.5	6	5	3	5.5
2,500	11	5.5	7	6.5	4	9
3,000	13	6	7	7	5	13

*Approximately 60% of calories from carbohydrate, 20% from protein, and 20% from fat for diets up to 2,000 kcal. For 2,500 and 3,000 kcal diets, ratios are approximately 56% carbohydrate, 19% protein, and 25% fat.
†If you eat a MEDIUM- or HIGH-FAT MEAT, or LOW-FAT or WHOLE MILK, be sure to account for the appropriate number of FAT exchanges.

find you must go lower to lose weight, decrease each exchange category proportionally and use a vitamin/mineral supplement.

HOW TO USE THE EXCHANGE SYSTEM

There are several advantages to using exchanges rather than counting calories: (a) the Exchange System enables you to balance your diet while cutting calories; (b) you can begin to think in terms of types of food and overall amounts instead of constantly counting calories; (c) you can easily adapt exchanges to meals served in restaurants; and (d) the system is adaptable to any number of daily caloric intakes.

Keep in mind, however, that part of the ease in using the Exchange System is that the values are approximate. You may look up an exchange item in a calorie guide and find that the caloric, carbohydrate, protein, and fat content don't exactly match for a given amount. Don't get hung up on this apparent discrepency; some exchanges are slight overestimates of nutrient content and some are slight underestimates. Overall, the calories and nutrients balance out.

An example of how to use the Exchange System is as follows:

Jane Dancer wants to eat a low-fat, balanced diet of 1,200 kcal a day. Table 7.1 tells her the number of exchanges she can consume under each of the six main food categories. Appendix A tells her the foods and amounts for each exchange. For a 1,200 kcal diet (in its simplest form), Jane can eat:

1. 4.5 STARCH exchanges (e.g., 4.5 slices of bread).
2. 3 LEAN MEAT exchanges (e.g., 3 oz of chicken without skin).
3. 5 VEGETABLE exchanges (e.g., 5 cups of raw vegetables).
4. 3 FRUIT exchanges (e.g., 3 small apples).
5. 2.5 SKIM MILK exchanges (e.g., 2½ cups of skim milk).
6. 3.5 FAT exchanges (e.g., 3½ tsp of butter or margarine).

Of course, this is a pretty boring diet because we have not used any variety in assigning the foods for each exchange group. However, Jane's FRUIT choices might include 1 apple, 1 banana, and some fruit sorbet, her STARCH exchanges might include pasta or muffins as well as bread, and so on. The timing of when she eats what foods is also up to Jane. The Exchange System provides a framework for a healthy diet, but the advantage is that *you* get to decide on the specifics.

When first using the Exchange System, you should measure out portions as precisely as you can. However, as you become more familiar with portion sizes, you can begin to visually estimate the amounts of certain items. The one category you should continue to measure is FAT because of the caloric density. A slight overestimate of FAT exchanges can add up to significant extra calories, whereas it is usually insignificant in the other categories.

CALCULATING EXCHANGES FROM NUTRITION LABELS

You can also assess the exchange value of any food that has its nutritional content printed on the package. For combination prepared foods, such as frozen dinners, the exchange values can be calculated from the label information on calories, protein, carbohydrate, and fat. (Many "light" frozen dinners even list the exchange values for you.) For example, "Chicken Étude," a frozen entrée, contains chicken, broccoli, carrots, and rice. The total number of calories is 260, with 20 grams of protein, 22 grams of carbohydrate, and 10 grams of fat. You can calculate the correct number of exchanges as follows:

1. A LEAN MEAT exchange contains 55 kcal, 7 grams of protein, and 3 grams of fat. Therefore, the number of LEAN MEAT exchanges for "Chicken Étude" will be between two and three. If we start with LEAN MEAT and assign 2.5 exchanges, we have accounted for 137.5 kcal, 17.5 grams of protein, and 7.5 grams of fat.

2. A STARCH exchange contains 80 kcal, 15 grams of carbohydrate, and 2 grams of protein; so the number of STARCH exchanges will be one or two. If we assign 1 STARCH exchange, we account for 80 kcal, 15 grams of carbohydrate, and 2 grams of protein.

3. A VEGETABLE exchange contains 25 kcal, 5 grams of carbohydrate, and 2 grams of protein. We have already accounted for 15 grams of carbohydrate with our STARCH exchange, so if we add one VEGETABLE exchange we will now have accounted for 20 grams of carbohydrate, just 2 short of the 22 grams included in "Chicken Étude."

4. A FAT exchange contains 45 kcal and 5 grams of fat. The number of FAT exchanges we assign to "Chicken Étude" will depend on how much fat is used up in the LEAN MEAT exchanges. Because we have already accounted for 7.5 grams of fat with our 2.5 LEAN MEAT exchanges, there are only 2.5 grams of fat left, which we account for with 0.5 FAT exchanges (22.5 kcal).

So, we now have calculated the following:

2.5 LEAN MEAT exchanges:	2.5 × 55 kcal =	137.5 kcal
1 STARCH exchanges:	1 × 80 kcal =	80.0 kcal
1 VEGETABLE exchanges:	1 × 25 kcal =	25.0 kcal
0.5 FAT exchanges:	0.5 × 45 kcal =	22.5 kcal
		255.0 kcal

When we add up all the protein grams for our exchanges we get 21.5 (remember to include those from STARCH and VEGETABLE categories as well as MEAT); our carbohydrate grams total 20; and our fat grams add up to 10. "Chicken Étude" actually contains 260 kcal, 20 grams of protein, 22 grams of carbohydrate, and 10 grams of fat; so our exchanges work out very well. Remember, exchange values are *approximate*. You need not try to get exact values with your calculations. (A list of sample frozen dinners and their exchange values is in Appendix B.)

Exhanges can also be combined to account for certain foods such as peanut butter (FAT and MEAT), cookies (STARCH and FAT), and ice cream (MILK, FRUIT, and FAT). Dessert foods need not be totally ruled out; in fact, it is probably wise to include some "goodie" foods in your plan to stave off total gustatory boredom. Examples of these foods and their exchange values are listed in Appendix C.

Turkey and chicken can be especially useful to the dancer in trying to consume high-protein, low-fat products. Table 7.3 gives the caloric and fat content of various poultry products.

PLANNING BY FOOD CATEGORY

As you do your initial diet planning, it may seem confusing counting up your exchanges. However, soon you will be able to design a diet schedule based on general food groups, and

Table 7.3. Caloric and Fat Content of Poultry Products

Type	Amount	Calories	Fat (g)
Skinless Turkey*			
Light meat	1 oz	45	1
Breast meat	1 oz	35	0.8
Dark meat	1 oz	55	2
Ground Turkey (dark, light, skin)	1 oz	65	4
Skinless Chicken*			
Light meat	1 oz	50	1.3
Breast meat	1 oz	40	0.9
Dark meat	1 oz	60	2.8
Turkey Cold Cuts			
Pastrami	1 oz	40	1.5
Ham	1 oz	35	1.5
Bologna	1 oz	60	5
Smoked Breast	1 oz	35	1.1
Frankfurter	1 (2 oz)	130	10

*Roasted or cooked without fat.
Source: Pennington, J. A., & Church, H. N. (1987). *Food Values of Portions Commonly Used*, Philadelphia: JB Lippincott.

not have to count every calorie. For example, think in terms of the following combinations:

- *Breakfast:* FRUIT, STARCH, MILK; e.g., fruit, cereal, skim milk.
- *Mid-Morning Snack:* MEAT, STARCH, FAT, FRUIT; e.g., cottage cheese, muffin, margarine, fruit juice.
- *Lunch:* VEG, MEAT, STARCH, FAT; e.g., green salad, tuna, bread, dressing.
- *Afternoon Snack:* MILK, VEG, STARCH or FRUIT; e.g., skim milk yogurt, raw vegetables, crackers or fresh fruit.
- *Dinner:* MEAT, VEG, FAT, STARCH, FRUIT; e.g., turkey, vegetables, salad, dressing, pasta, dessert fruit.
- *Evening Snack:* Optional; e.g., skim milk or yogurt, or cottage cheese, or 1 tsp peanut butter. (Milk products and peanut butter have high levels of tryptophan, an amino acid precursor to serotonin, which promotes relaxation. Peanut butter has a high fat content, however.)

The spacing of food consumption into three small meals and three snacks leads us into our next discussion: why it is important *not* to go too long without eating.

What to Eat and When to Eat

Traditionally, dieters have been told they should eat only when they are hungry, and dancers often try to abstain from eating for long periods. This may sound good but for most people, especially dancers, waiting until hunger is strong can actually have an *adverse* affect on your metabolism. Much of the reason involves the hormone insulin and how it can respond after long periods without food.

Insulin is a key hormone in the regulation of blood glucose (sugar) and works to *lower* blood glucose levels by (a) increasing diffusion of glucose into muscle and fat cells; (b) promoting storage of glucose as glycogen in the liver and muscle cells; and (c) enhancing the uptake of glucose by fat and liver cells for conversion into fat. Basically, insulin helps "feed" blood glucose to muscle, liver, and fat cells.

Normally, insulin levels peak about 30–60 minutes after eating, initiating the transfer of glucose from the blood into muscle, liver, and fat cells. Insulin levels usually peak at the same time blood glucose levels are at their peak, so there is plenty of blood glucose to be "fed" to the cells. However, after long periods without food, four to six hours, the insulin response can "overshoot" and cause blood glucose levels to drop dramatically. This is often followed by a craving for carbohydrates, which is, in part, the body's response to the low blood glucose levels.

The response of insulin to blood glucose is one of a number of factors that determine how hungry you get. Therefore, it is wise to try to avoid the large swings in blood sugar that result from hours of not eating.

It is important to work out a schedule of consistent food intake throughout the day to avoid potentially large swings in blood glucose levels. Eating small amounts of foods containing protein, carbohydrate, and fat about every three hours can help avoid low blood sugar and the resultant "low-blood sugar jitters." In general, simple sugars should be avoided because of the abrupt insulin response, as well as caffeine because it indirectly lowers blood glucose levels through stimulation of the hormone epinephrine. Alcohol should also be avoided because it can block *gluconeogenesis* (conversion of protein into glucose). And, believe it or not, sugar substitutes should also be avoided in view of the fact that some nutritionists feel they may trigger an insulin response.

One of the most common complaints we hear regarding eating numerous small meals comes from those dancers who find it difficult to tolerate breakfast. Many say they just feel sick in morning class if they eat before hand, or else that they feel hungrier throughout the day if they eat breakfast. Yet, we know blood sugar levels can be adversely affected if night time fasting continues too long into the day. Dancers with this problem should try avoiding caffeine in the morning (yes, it can be done) and eating a light snack about 45 minutes before class—perhaps yogurt, fruit, and cereal. After class, another similar snack should be consumed, with the rest of the day's meals consisting of lunch, mid-afternoon snack, dinner, and evening snack. If, after trying this for awhile, the before-class light meal is still a problem, plan a more substantial meal for after class. Remember, going more than four or five waking hours without food may ultimately result in an overconsumption of carbohydrates.

Preperformance Meals

Another big question concerning timing of meals is with regard to performance. Most experienced performers have developed their own eating routine prior to performance, but some general guidelines are offered for those who have not established such a routine or who would like to improve their current one.

The main factors that influence the optimal sequence between eating and performance are timing and meal composition. Ideally, food should have passed through the stomach and upper intestines by performance time. Digestion time depends on both the amount and type of food consumed, as well as factors such as emotional tension. Fasting prior to performance is not recommended, however. Studies on runners have demonstrated that fasting 12–24 hours prior to activity is detrimental to performance (Sherman, 1989).

The preperformance meal should consist primarily of complex carbohydrates. Fructose (fruit sugar) should only be consumed in combination with other carbohydrates because fructose alone can cause gastric upset. Foods high in fat and protein should also be avoided because they tend to keep food in the stomach and upper intestine, and can trigger an increase in the acidity of the blood. Other foods to avoid include those high in salt (potato chips, canned soups), fiber (bran products), and those that tend to produce gas (lettuce, beans, raw vegetables). Your best bets for preperformance foods are pasta, whole grain breads, cereal, fruit, and yogurt.

Most studies of preperformance meals have been conducted on endurance athletes, so we don't have much information on how meals affect a high-intensity interval activity like dance. However, you may wish to consider the following guidelines to get grams of carbohydrate you should consume prior to a performance (adapted from Sherman, 1989):

1. One hour prior to performance: Body Weight in pounds × .45 = grams of carbohydrate.

2. Two to three hours prior: Body Weight × .90 (female), or 1.1 (male) = grams of carbohydrate.
3. Four hours prior: Body Weight × 1.8 (female), or 2.25 (male) = grams of carbohydrate.

For example, a 110 lb female dancer consumes her preperformance meal at 7 p.m, for an 8 p.m. curtain. 110 lb × .45 = 49.5 grams of carbohydrate, so her meal consists of:

Serving/Food	Carbohydrate
1 whole banana	30 grams
1 slice whole wheat bread	15 grams
1 tsp fruit jam or jelly	4 grams
	49 grams

If this same dancer opted to eat her meal two to three hours before curtain (between 5:00 and 6:00 p.m.), she would plan for 99 grams of carbohydrate (110 lb × .90 = 99). If she found that her best regimen was to eat four hours prior to performance, at 4:00 p.m., she would consume 198 grams of carbohydrate (110 lb × 1.8 = 198). Other good carbohydrate choices include:

Serving/Food	Carbohydrate
8 oz fruit-flavored low-fat yogurt	40–46 grams
1 cup unsweetened apple sauce	30 grams
2 cups cooked pasta	60–80 grams
1/2 cup spaghetti sauce	20 grams
2 Tbsp raisins	15–20 grams

Remember, these are only guidelines. Every individual responds differently and not every performance has the same energy requirements. Some dancers may need to augment their preperformance meals with protein if they have a particularly sensitive insulin response. If you find this for yourself, be sure the protein is very low in fat, such as skinless chicken or turkey breast, or small amounts of 1 percent cottage cheese. Yogurt is a good choice because it supplies some protein but is easily digestible.

It is very important that each dancer initially test the effectiveness of preperformance meals and timing during rehearsal, *not* prior to a major production. Overall weight control efforts may need to be adjusted according to carbo-hydrate needs during periods of frequent performance.

Cravings

Almost any dancer who has tried various methods of weight control eventually comes up against what we call "killer cravings." These are not just the ordinary "Gee, that cheese-cake looks good" attractions we all feel occasionally. These are the overwhelming "If I don't get some chocolate (or whatever), I'm going to die" urges that are often accompa-nied by feeling nervous and sometimes even lightheaded. Women usually report such cravings prior to their periods.

Although no one really knows the mechanism of these cravings, current evidence points to hormonal-chemical interactions. For example, the majority of women who report having cravings prior to their periods say it is specific to chocolate. Not just sugar, not just fat, but chocolate. This has led some researchers to believe that a chemical in chocolate, theobromine, may react with the female hormone progesterone.

But the question is, what do you *do* about cravings when the food you crave is fattening? There are two main schools of thought in response to this: One says to avoid the craved item and focus on larger quantities other, healthier foods. The other school recommends consuming a small amount of the object of your craving as soon as you notice it.

Here's how one dancer we know handles the situation: "I always know when my period is due because I get an intense craving for chocolate exactly 24 hours beforehand. I used to try everything to avoid eating chocolate but ended up overeating all kinds of other things, and then would often give into the chocolate craving anyway. Finally I tried eating a small amount of chocolate the minute I felt the urge, like maybe ¼ or ½ a chocolate bar, along with a glass of skim milk. I found the chocolate satisfied the craving and the milk kept me from overindulging. After this, I try to go for a walk or do some other type of exercise, which also seems to help."

Milk chocolate contains about 150 kcal per oz, 2 grams protein, 16 grams carbohydrate, and 9 grams fat (1 FRUIT, 2 FAT exchanges). (One ounce is equal to about six Her-shey's Kisses.) If you're subject to premenstrual chocolate cravings, you may wish to try the method described above by consuming ½ oz of chocolate and 4 oz of skim milk (40 kcal, 4 grams protein, 6 grams carbohydrate, no fat) for a total of 115 kcal, 5 grams protein, 14 grams of carbohydrate, and 4.5 grams fat (½ SKIM MILK, ½ FRUIT, 1 FAT exchanges).

Food Intake versus Energy Expenditure

In trying to determine the number of calories for your total food intake, basic energy requirements and additional expenditures need to be considered. Although individual differences in metabolic rate affect such determinations, you can get a general idea of where to set your food intake goals in terms of weight management.

First, you need to consider "basal energy expenditure" (BEE), which is the energy needed to sustain the body in a resting state. The equation includes weight, height, and age:

Equation for estimating BEE (Krause & Mahan, 1984, p. 15):

Females: 655 + 9.6 (wt in kg)* + 1.85 (ht in cm) − 4.7 (age) = *BEE*

Males: 66.5 + 13.7 (wt in kg) + 5 (ht in cm) − 6.8 (age) = *BEE*

Example: A 25-year-old female weighs 120 lb and is 64 in. tall. To convert from pounds to kilograms and inches to centimeters see metric conversion tables, Appendix E and calculate as follows:

120 lb × .45 = 54 kg
64 in. × 2.54 = 163 cm

Use these values in the BEE equation to get:

655 + 9.6(*54 kg*) + 1.85(*163cm*) − 4.7(*25 yrs*) = 1,357

This dancer needs about 1,350 kcals a day for the body to sustain resting metabolism. Functional activities such as bathing, shopping, and walking would add about 20 percent, or 267 kcal, to this figure. Dancing would add about 200 kcal for every hour of dance where the activity is similar to an

---

*Bracket values are multiplied.

average 60-minute technique class. Add about 400–500 kcal for every hour of continuous aerobic exercise.

So, if our dancer carried out her normal daily activities as well as the kind of dance activity common to class and rehearsal for six hours, her energy demands would be about 2,850 kcal. Yet, as we discussed in Chapter 4, most dancers sustain their weight consuming far less than this. Why is this?

The problem has to do with the lowering of basal energy expenditure in response to diminished food intake—our old problem of adaptation. As food intake decreases, the body becomes more efficient. Many diet books fail to take this into account and consequently overestimate appropriate levels of caloric intake for weight loss. Basal energy expenditure is also why exercise is so important in weight control. Exercise helps maintain muscle tissue, which helps keep basal energy expenditure up.

Therefore, the BEE equation is intended to help you determine a basic caloric intake level to use with our balanced diet programs. Our recommendation is to calculate BEE for your *desired* weight, and then choose the diet plan reflecting that caloric value. For example, let's say our 25-year-old, 120 lb female wants to lose 10 lb and weigh 110. She replaces her original value of 54 kg with 50 kg in the BEE equation:

$$655 + 9.6(50 \ kg) + 1.85(163 \ cm) - 4.7(25yrs) = 1,319$$

Her weight-loss energy calculation for 110 lb is 1,319 kcal, so she can plan her diet for between 1,300 and 1,350 kcal. However, because of individual differences in basal metabolic rate, she may have to adjust her plan according to her own weight-loss response and energy needs.

In the next chapter, we will provide guidelines for aerobic exercise to promote fat and weight loss. We cannot overemphasize that dietary and exercise guidelines are intended to go together in a total health and weight management program.

Chapter VIII Guidelines on Endurance Exercise to Burn Fat

As discussed in Chapter 2, not all aerobic exercise promotes fat utilization. Although aerobic exercise is any activity that can be done continuously at a heart rate of 70–80 percent of maximum for 12–20 minutes, *endurance* aerobic exercise involves at least 30 minutes of activity at a heart rate of 60–70 percent of maximum. During moderate-duration aerobic exercise, the body will burn some fat but will rely primarily on glucose as its fuel source. In contrast, endurance aerobic exercise causes the body to use fat as its primary fuel source because of the lower levels of intensity and longer durations involved. The longer the duration, the more fat is burned.

For a dancer who is currently in good dance condition, use the following guidelines to calculate heart rate for endurance exercise:

Multiply your age-predicted max heart rate by .60 and .65. Example for a 21-year-old:

$$220 - 21 = 199 \text{ bpm (age-predicted max)}$$
$$199 \times .60 = 119 \text{ bpm}$$
$$199 \times .65 = 129 \text{ bpm}$$

So, in order to exercise at a level that will burn primarily fats as fuel, this dancer should exercise 30 minutes or longer at a heart rate of between about 120 and 130 bpm. The minimum duration should be 30 minutes because it takes at least this long for the hormonal releases which promote fat utilization to occur.

If you are not currently in good overall dance condition, start off by using .50 and .60 to determine your endurance heart rate range. We make this recommendation because of the possibility of musculoskeletal injury if you start out at an endurance rate that is too high relative to your condition.

You may have also heard the term "target heart rate" used in conjunction with aerobic conditioning. Be aware that what we have just presented is *not* the same as target heart rate.

Working at your target heart rate will involve a more intense energy output, which, while excellent for training the heart muscle and cardiovascular system, will cause the body to use glucose as its primary fuel source rather than fat. However, to *improve* cardiovascular condition, target heart rate must be maintained during a 15–20 minute workout. General target heart rate is about 70 percent of agepredicted maximum heart rate.

Individual target heart rate is determined by the equation:

[(Max Heart Rate − Resting Heart Rate) × .60] + Resting Heart Rate = Target Heart Rate

If our 21-year-old has a resting heart rate of 63 bpm, her target heart rate is: [(199 bpm − 63 bpm) × .60] + 63 bpm = 144 bpm. This is higher than what is recommended for endurance exercise.

We realize that all this can sound confusing, but here's where the apparent conflict lies. In training to make *improvements* in your fitness level, the heart must be worked harder than what is ideal to promote fat utilization. However, the greater your fitness level, the more fat you burn during exercise. Sound like a contradiction? Well, it all has to do with training the body to break down fat more readily and also promote fat loss. The fact of the matter is, one should combine exercise that improves fitness and promotes fat utilization.

For example, our 21-year-old dancer wants to start an aerobic exercise program. She feels she is in good shape as far as dance goes but has never really tried any aerobic exercise. She starts out with a 15-minute workout on an exercise bicycle, working at her target heart rate in an attempt to improve her cardiovascular fitness (about 144 bpm or 70 percent of maximum). She feels like she has gotten a fair workout with this but thinks she can do more, so the next day she decides to ride 30 minutes at the same intensity. This time, her legs begin to feel like lead after about 10 minutes, and after 15 minutes she has to stop. She wonders why this felt so easy the first day but was so difficult the second. The answer lies in a concept known as "specific adaptation to imposed demands," or the SAID principle.

The SAID Principle

The SAID principle applies to all activities and means simply that the body will respond specifically, both muscularly and cardiovascularly, to the *specific* type of training demanded of it. So, even though our dancer is well-conditioned for the specific muscular and cardiovascular demands of dance, her body is not prepared to operate in a well-conditioned manner in something like cycling. The muscles that must repeatedly contract in the cycling motion do not work in the same way as those used for dance. Also, as a dancer, she is conditioned for short bursts of activity. That type of *interval* work is very different from the *continuous* work demanded by 15 minutes of steady cycling.

The first day our dancer exercised, adrenaline and psychological freshness allowed her body to function fairly well during the cycling. But the second day, as muscle soreness and fatigue began to set in, the true picture emerged. If she wants to continue her cycling program, she will have to train her body to adapt to the specific demands of cycling. This is done the same way one trains for anything: by gradually increasing the duration and intensity of the exercise.

Sample Exercise Program to Promote Fat Loss

Using the SAID principle, our dancer revamps her exercise program to gradually accommodate longer workouts and build her fitness level. The entire program, with recommended times and heart rates, is presented in Chart 8.1. Any appropriate activity can be used, but we recommend something that is low-impact (such as walking) or non-weight bearing (such as cycling).

Chart 8.1 lists total exercise time and interval times. Interval sets are repeated until the total time is completed. For example, Week 1/Day 1 starts off at 15 minutes, with intervals of 3 minutes at 60 percent max heart rate and 2 minutes at 70 percent max heart rate. The interval set is 5 minutes (3 min + 2 min), which is repeated three times for a total 15-minute workout. For the 17 minute bout on Day 3, simply add one 2-minute interval after the third set repetition. Later on, in Week 7, the intervals involve continuous exercise at a given heart rate for 10 minutes or more, and interval sets are not repeated.

Chart 8.1. Exercise Guidelines for Dancers to Promote Body Fat Loss

	Day 1	Day 2	Day 3	Day 4	Day 5	Day 6	Day 7
Wk 1	15 min* 3 min 60%† 2 min 70% 3 reps§	Repeat Day 1.1	17 min 3 min 60% 2 min 70% 3.5 reps	Rest	Repeat Day 1.3	20 min 3 min 60% 2 min 70% 4 reps	Rest
Wk 2	20 min 3 min 60% 2 min 70% 4 reps	Repeat Day 2.1	23 min 3 min 60% 2 min 70% 4.5 reps	Rest	Repeat Day 2.3	25 min 3 min 65% 2 min 75% 5 reps	Rest
Wk 3	Rest	Depends on con- dition	25 min 3 min 60% 2 min 70% 5 reps	Rest	Repeat Day 3.3	30 min 3 min 65% 2 min 75% 6 reps	Rest
Wk 4	30 min 3 min 60% 2 min 70% 6 reps	Repeat Day 4.1	33 min 3 min 60% 2 min 70% 6.5 reps	Rest	Repeat Day 4.3	35 min 3 min 65% 2 min 80% 7 reps	Rest
Wk 5	35 min 3 min 60% 2 min 70% 7 reps	Repeat Day 5.1	40 min 3 min 60% 2 min 70% 8 reps	Rest	Repeat Day 5.3	45 min 3 min 60% 2 min 70% 9 reps	Rest
Wk 6	45 min 3 min 60% 2 min 70% 9 reps	Repeat Day 6.1	48 min 3 min 60% 2 min 70% 9.5 reps	Rest	Repeat Day 6.3	50 min 3 min 60% 2 min 70% 10 reps	Rest
Wk 7	50 min 10 min 70% 20 min 65% 20 min 60%	Repeat Day 7.1	53 min 10 min 70% 20 min 65% 23 min 60%	Rest	Repeat Day 7.3	55 min 10 min 70% 20 min 65% 25 min 60%	Rest
Wk 8	55 min 10 min 70% 20 min 65% 25 min 60%	Repeat Day 8.1	58 min 10 min 70% 20 min 65% 28 min 60%	Rest	Repeat Day 8.3	60 min 10 min 70% 20 min 65% 30 min 60%	Rest

Subsequent weeks should follow general guidelines of 30 to 60 minutes, 4 to 5 days a week, at 60% of max heartrate until body comp goals are reached. Maintenance exercise should include 30 to 4 minutes, 3 days a week, at 60 to 65% max HR.

*Total Exercise Time.
†Interval Time, % max HR.
§Repetitions of interval set.

GENERAL EXERCISE GUIDELINES:

• **Each exercise bout should be preceded by a 5-minute warm-up.** Stretching alone is not warm-up. Warm-up should involve large, easy, repetitive motions of all body joints that slowly increase the body temperature. Warm-up is *not* included in the total exercise time.

• **Each exercise bout should conclude with a 5-minute cool-down.** This is basically the reverse of warm-up, allowing for a gradual decrease in body temperature. If you wish to stretch to increase or maintain flexibility, it is best to do so as part of the cool-down phase. Stretching is better facilitated by the increased body temperature resulting from activity. Intense stretching prior to exercise bouts such as these may actually be detrimental due to possible interference with reflexive mechanisms that protect against injury. Cool-down is not included in the total exercise time.

• **Adequate water intake should be maintained during the exercise bout.** Drinking 3–4 ounces of water every 10–15 minutes should prevent dehydration. After the bout, more water should be consumed, approximately 8 ounces for every 30 minutes of exercise.

• **Adequate rest days should be incorporated into any exercise plan.** This is *very* important. Rest allows for recovery of stressed tissue, which is a crucial part of training. Without it you take one step back for every two steps forward. Rest, however, does not mean doing nothing. It simply means *not* doing the training activity.

Exercise Induced Anemia

Even with adequate rest days, it is common to get to the 14-day point in a new training regimen and, without warning, suddenly feel like you've been hit by a truck. This common occurrence is generally due to what is known as "exercise induced anemia." In this condition, the production of hemoglobin, the oxygen carrying molecule in the blood, gradually falls behind in terms of supply-and-demand. With the increase in exercise, greater amounts of oxygen must be transported and more hemoglobin is needed to do so. The body makes hemoglobin at a rate usually sufficient to keep up with demand, but as exercise continues, the production of hemoglobin can fall short. Why it happens at the 14-day point is anybody's guess, but it does so with amazing regularity.

Generally people suffering from exercise induced anemia feel crummy for a few days and begin to wonder if all the exercise is worth it. (This is also the point at which many people throw in the towel on their weight-loss programs.) Should you just try to muscle through this period and stay on your exercise schedule? No, it is better to cut back and let the body rebuild its hemoglobin. This is only a temporary situation, and running the body past its limits will only lead to more fatigue.

Heart Rates and Types of Activity

The program presented in Chart 8.1 involves gradually building up cardiovascular fitness using interval training, and at the same time working to increase endurance time. This program is designed for dancers, who generally already have good levels of cardiovascular fitness. The heart rates are therefore higher than those appropriate for untrained individuals. To measure your heart rate while exercising, it is best to take your radial artery pulse, which is just to the thumb side of the prominent tendons on the palmar surface of the wrist. You can also take your carotid artery pulse, which is just to either side of your "Adam's Apple" in the throat. However, if you use the carotid pulse, press very lightly because the vagus nerve runs right along this area. The vagus nerve helps regulate heart rate and is very sensitive to pressure. Pressing too hard may artificially speed up or slow down your heart rate. Never use the thumb for pulse taking since there is already a weak pulse in that area.

After eight weeks of her exercise program, our dancer should be able to determine what is working best. She may wish to increase the duration of her workout, she may wish to return to some interval training, or she may just stick with a steady-state, 60-minute workout, keeping her heart rate at about 60 percent of max.

Other examples of activities that are appropriate for long-duration exercise and that promote fat losses include walking, jogging, aerobic dance, crosscountry skiing (or using a machine that simulates the motion), and rowing (not recommended as it is hard on the back). Even dance movements may be done continuously for an hour as endurance exercise, as long as the duration and intensity conditions are met. The one exception is swimming. Even though swimming can be done in an endurance fashion, recent research has demonstrated that swimming does not promote fat loss the same way walking or jogging does (Gwinup, 1987). The reasons for this are not entirely clear, but it may have something to do with the lower body temperature in swimming as compared to other sports.

Once you have reached your body composition goal, exercise frequency can be reduced to 30-minute bouts, three to four times a week. Again, this exercise program should be combined with the dietary modifications suggested in Chapter 7 in order to promote desired changes in your body composition.

When Will I Start Losing Weight?

One of the barriers to continuing a balanced diet and exercise program is that you don't see the kind of immediate drops in weight that you do on traditional crash diets. However, keep in mind that any daily changes in weight of more than a pound are due to *water* loss or gain, not fat. In fact, be forewarned that in starting an endurance exercise program, you may not see any weight loss for a week or two, and might even see a slight gain. There are a couple of reasons for this. One is that glycogen stores build up in response to increases in exercise, and with the increased glycogen comes an increase in water. Another reason is the maintenance of muscle mass with exercise (remember, starvation dieting results in the burning of muscle tissue during the first three to seven days). True fat losses take longer to show up on the scale than water or muscle loss.

Naturally, this can be very discouraging but it is important to stick with your long-term plan. Once these initial physiologic adaptations take place, the body gears itself toward fat burning and will start showing the kinds of changes you want. Bear in mind that you can replace a pound of fat with a pound of muscle and still end up with a smaller body.

One way you can assess your own progress is with "the jeans test." Dig out an old pair of jeans that are too tight and try them on once a week. As one dancer put it, "The jeans will tell you that good things are happening before your scale or measuring tape will." On a low-fat, reduced calorie diet and endurance exercise program, you will start seeing weight and body composition changes in about three to six weeks. We know this sounds slow, but the point is that these methods constitute a long-term *investment* in weight control rather than a quick gamble.

Physical Considerations: Avoiding Injury

Many of you may be thinking, "I dance eight hours a day as it is, how am I going to put in *another* hour of exercise to lose weight?" This is certainly an important consideration and one that should not be taken lightly. All the best intentions can result in even more frustration if during the first week of your new exercise program you sustain an injury that keeps you out of both exercise and dance.

The main consideration when adding more activity to your dance schedule is the degree of weight-bearing impact required. That is, will the new activity require repetitive jumping or similar activity that might overstress the body? Activities such as jogging or high-impact aerobics come with a high risk of injury, and for this reason, dancers may wish to avoid these in favor of other less impact-loading ventures. Low-impact aerobics are a good alternative if the instructor is certified by the American College of Sports Medicine (ACSM). Many fitness clubs advertise that their instructors are certified, but the certifications may be in-house and therefore not a good indicator of the instructor's expertise. Ask before you pay.

Sometimes low-impact aerobics do not avail themselves to the type of training that promotes fat loss and increases in cardiovascular fitness. One study found that a 10-minute, low-impact workout resulted in a heart rate 11 bpm less than a comparable high-impact sequence. If you find your heart rate does not go high enough during a low-impact class, try using a weighted vest or belt. (Hand weights have not been proven effective in increasing energy demands.) Any added weight should be kept close to the body's center of gravity, where it is less likely to cause joint injuries. You may also be able to secure ankle weights around your waist if they have extended velcro fasteners. Start off with 3–5 lb of added weight and see if this results in a higher heart rate. If it does not, gradually add more weight, but for safety, do not exceed 10 lb.

Long-duration walking is another activity which is less stressful on the body than running, and added weight around the center of the body can be useful here as well. Weights should *never* be worn on the ankles during weight bearing exercise. Damage to ligaments of the knee is one of the serious risks of doing so. (Ankle weights can be safely used for controlled strengthening exercises, however.)

Even a low-impact workout does not mean you are immune to injury. Recalling the SAID principle, every new activity you start will require a new adaptation to its specific demands. New stresses on tendons and ligaments can cause problems even if repetitive pounding is not involved. In order to minimize the possibility of injury, *any* new activity, even dance movements done in an aerobic fashion, must be approached with a gradual, systematic build-up of intensity. We strongly advise that you *do not exceed* the weekly workout times outlined in Chart 8.1. If anything, you may wish to be more conservative.

You should also pay close attention to your body's warning signs. If you feel unduly sore or stiff in a particular area of your body after beginning your exercise program, consider cutting back on the time or intensity. Be sure your rest days are really rest days and if need be, take an extra one if you feel you are on the verge of overdoing it.

If you do experience injury, immediately apply ice to the injured part for approximately 20 minutes and repeat once every hour or two for the first 24 hours after the injury (except when asleep). If you have injured a knee or ankle, elevate the injured joint to a point that is higher than your heart. If it is a back injury, the ice rule still applies. Any injury, whether it is a muscle strain, a ligament sprain, or a "back spasm" (which is usually the result of a strain or sprain), involves inflammation. Ice reduces inflammation as well as injury due to secondary tissue death from lack of oxygen to the affected site. Heat increases blood flow to the area and therefore increases the metabolic rate, which you don't want to occur during the initial phases of an injury. You want to *decrease* the metabolic rate of the area in order to minimize the secondary damage. When in doubt, ice. If the injury does not improve within 48 hours, be sure to see a physician, physical therapist, or certified athletic trainer.

The Importance of Drinking Water

Every chemical reaction in your body is dependent on one common substance: water. Without adequate hydration (drinking enough water), the body cannot carry out the tremendous energy expenditures we ask of it without sacrifice. That sacrifice is usually in the form of muscle spasm, fatigue, and possible kidney damage.

Water is one substance dancers can ingest without worrying about calories or side-effects, assuming it's "good" water.* Yet many dancers overlook this simple and effective way of improving their health, body composition, and energy status.

In our study of dancers (Chmelar et al., 1987) we found the majority (54 percent) had very poor levels of water intake. Our subjects depended heavily on caffeine-containing diet drinks and coffee, and many said they drank only one or two full glasses of plain water a day.

Dancers should consume at least 64 oz of water, or about eight full glasses, each day. Contrary to what some may say, you won't get "bloated" by increasing water intake. The body's fluid levels are maintained by a hormonal feedback mechanism and by consuming adequate amounts of water, you will actually aid your body in dispensing fluid wastes. A simple way to determine if you are maintaining an adequate water intake is to weigh yourself before and after a day of classes and/or rehearsal. You should drink enough fluid to keep your morning and after work-out weights equal.

The practice of wearing plastic "sauna" pants or of sweating in a real sauna will only dehydrate the body—*no fat is lost.* Many dancers resort to these methods the day before a weigh-in. It is unfortunate that companies and dance departments may play a part in promoting such practices, however unintentionally. If you are in such a situation and do find yourself dehydrated, be sure to replenish your fluid levels as quickly as possible.

*An exception involves water intoxication, which is covered in "Other Eating Disorders Issues" in Chapter 9.

Scheduling an Exercise Program

Many dancers find their schedules during performance seasons are so packed that engaging in an extra hour of exercise five days a week leaves them exhausted and unable to keep up with the demands of performing. Again, this is an important consideration, but it does not mean there are no alternatives.

First of all, your exercise program does not have to be done in an all-or-none fashion. If you can only tolerate 20 minutes, three times a week, it can certainly be of benefit when combined with low-fat dietary modifications. Also, most dancers have periods during the year when dance demands are relatively low. These slow periods for dance can be used as an excellent time to start a weight-loss exercise program.

In fact, taking some time off from intense dancing and switching to an aerobic activity may be just the boost a dancer needs in order to get her weight modification program off to a good start. There are both physical and psychological advantages to this approach. Physically, the body needs time to recover from months of any intense activity, and dance is certainly intense. While the repetitive motions of dance are important for building strength and coordination, they can also result in overuse injuries if adequate recovery time is not incorporated into training. However, in order to recover one does not need complete rest. Total lack of activity can actually be detrimental to the dancer in that fitness levels and muscle tone are sacrificed at the expense of recovery. A change of activity, on the other hand, can be beneficial because joints and muscle patterns overused in dance can recover while the dancer maintains his or her general fitness level.

As for psychological benefits, breaks from dance can help prevent burn-out and also allow time for fresh insights into dance to develop. How many times have you had a difficult problem that you forgot about for a few days, only to then find that the solution to the problem had become obvious? A similar pattern can occur in dance both physically and psychologically when a nondance activity is practiced.

In order to promote weight-loss, the alternative nondance activity should be endurance aerobic according to the guidelines we have presented. It should also involve whole-body, full range-of-motion movements that do not pose a serious threat of injury. Basic strength and flexibility should be maintained and the activity should be relatively easy on joint compression. For example, weight training alone would not be a good alternative (for weight loss) whereas a walk-jog program would. One may also wish to combine activities, such as endurance walking and tai-chi, a nonaerobic, meditative activity. Return to dance classes and rehearsals after your break should be planned well in advance to avoid the physical shock of returning to the highly specified demands of dance. Before you are scheduled to return to your university or company classes, gradually rebuild your dance activity by starting some barre or floor work either on your own or in a nondemanding organized situation.

We realize these recommendations go against the generally accepted advice to *never* take more than a week off from dancing; however, we have found that giving your body and mind a rest from the intricate demands of dance may be the best thing you can do to prolong your dance life and attain your body composition goals.

As most of us know, however, weight control is more than just what you eat and how much you exercise. Just as psychological factors play an important role in dance training and performance, so do they play a crucial role in weight management, which we will discuss in Chapter 9.

Chapter IX

Psychological Factors and Eating Disorders

Psychological Factors

Theories of weight control have run the gamut from those based primarily on psychological factors to those based mainly on physiological factors. Many studies have shown that people who diet regularly exhibit altered psychological patterns, but the question remains as to whether the dieting is a *cause* or a *result* of these changes in mental outlook.

For dancers, the deck is already stacked because of the low body-weight requirements of the profession. The psychological pressures on dancers are therefore not the same as those on the average young woman who is responding to societal expectations to be thin. Most dancers must be thin to continue their careers, which is very different from wanting to be thin for social reasons.

It is important to differentiate the psychological responses of a dancer working diligently toward career goals and someone who is obsessed with body weight because of problems with self-esteem or other internal conflicts. The distinction is blurry, to be sure, but the fact is that while dancers may appear to be merely obsessed with weight and body image, this "obsession" is directed by the demands of their profession. In other words, it comes with the job and is not necessarily a negative psychological trait, although it can become one. (For a more detailed discussion of the psychology of dance and body image, we refer the reader to the work of L. M. Vincent and Suzanne Gordon listed in the bibliography, as well as the specific research articles listed on this subject.)

In attempting to modify your body composition, the interdependence of physiology and psychology should not be underestimated. As food intake is diminished, psychological changes can occur in response. Also, as personal and professional problems arise, the body can respond with physiologic changes in appetite. Therefore, it is important to maintain a balanced perspective regarding the inevitable ups and downs of your weight modification program.

One of the most common psychological problems for dancers attempting to lose weight are vast swings in self-esteem related to eating, i.e., "when I don't eat and lose weight, I'm perfect" vs. "when I eat and gain weight, I'm scum." These views ultimately gear the dancer toward failure and should be dealt with as part of any weight-modification program. The dancer may wish to keep a diary of emotional responses toward food, body weight, and dance in order to identify problem areas. The goal should be to ease the response on both ends of the spectrum so that changes in body weight are not exclusively connected with success or failure as a dancer.

Some studies indicate that the degree of social support a person receives while involved in a weight-loss attempt is particularly important. One problem in the dance world is that successful weight loss and competition with other dancers can be intimately connected. It may be difficult to receive support in an arena where many female dancers vie for relatively few choice company positions or roles. However, one of the most successful methods of providing psychological counseling and support is through organized peer groups. Getting together with other dancers facing similar weight modification challenges to discuss problems, feelings, and ways of overcoming common stumbling blocks can help build positive coping mechanisms and ease frustration. The important element in peer-support organizations is that possible solutions to problems be generated from within.

Not all dancers, however, will benefit from a group situation. Many may feel that such a group is just another pressure in the whole area of weight modification and feel they would do better on a solo plan. The important issue is that dancers try to recognize those emotional and psychological factors that might be influencing their eating behavior and take action to deal with them in a positive manner. Some may argue that dancers will just continue to deceive themselves about their eating habits unless they submit to professional therapy. However, we feel that most dancers have a great capacity for self-insight and that as long as the atmosphere is conducive to such explorations, the majority of dancers will be able to make positive self-discoveries.

We realize many may be thinking "But what about dancers with eating disorders? Shouldn't they seek professional counseling?" *Absolutely.* The above recommendations apply to those dancers who struggle with weight management but do not fall into the eating-disorders category. It is important, however, that directors, instructors, or friends dealing with a dancer who appears to be exhibiting signs of eating-disordered behavior be able to recognize those signs and take the appropriate steps in helping that dancer receive proper treatment.

Recognizing the Signs of Eating Disorders

Physical and behavioral signs that may indicate anorexia include: (a) excessive weight loss; (b) fine downy hair covering the body; (c) dry skin; (d) muscle atrophy; (e) refusal to ingest food; (f) distended abdomen; and (g) expressions of being "fat" despite continued weight loss.

Signs that may indicate bulimia include: (a) a continued "bloated" look despite minimal or no changes in weight; (b) yellowing and decay of the teeth (from repeated vomiting); (c) enlargement of salivary glands; (d) erratic eating patterns, i.e., consumption of large meals contrasted with long periods of eating nothing; and (e) change in skin tone, or appearance of dry and scaly skin. Be aware that physical signs may not be apparent until the eating-disordered behavior is well-established, and also that these signs may be indicative of other diseases.

Any dancer suspected of having an eating disorder should be approached with concern and caution, with the understanding that you are dealing with a potentially volatile situation. If you are the director of a professional or university program, become familiar with referral sources for treatment of eating disorders and be ready to discuss them with your dancers. If you find you must confront someone because of a probable eating disorder, it is best to consult an eating disorders professional beforehand on how to approach the situation. Despite good intentions, confrontations can do more harm than good if handled improperly.

Most states have medical treatment referral centers listed under "Physicians" in the Yellow Pages. Another good place to try is any major university-affiliated hospital in your area (ask for psychological counseling services and explain that it is an eating disorders problem).

Research on Eating Disorders and Dancers

The complexity of eating disorders is something that can only be justly handled in a full volume dedicated solely to that topic. Although we can hardly begin to address the many controversies, theories, and problems associated with this issue in a few short pages, we can discuss some of the research focusing specifically on eating disorders and dancers in an effort to promote better recognition of the problem.

There is a fuzzy distinction between what is considered to be obsession with thinness and what qualifies for anorexia nervosa. While anorexia nervosa has traditionally been defined as a disease of psychiatric origin, recent investigations of anorexia among dancers point to other important factors in the development of this disorder. Similarly, the development of bulimia may be more related to specific dieting behavior than to pre-existing psychological characteristics.

Linda Hamilton, J. Brooks-Gunn, and Michelle Warren have conducted extensive research into the area of eating disorders among female ballet dancers and while a complete review of their work is a must for anyone interested in this complicated subject, for our purposes we will highlight some of their major findings.*

Over the course of several studies (Hamilton et al., 1988; Hamilton et al., 1986; Hamilton et al., 1985), these researchers observed that eating disorders among ballet dancers were specifically related to three major areas: (a) ethnic/sociocultural influences; (b) competitive atmosphere of the dancer's environment; and (c) genetic influences on body weight. They also observed specific differences among those

---

*We know of no studies on eating disorders in male dancers, but it is estimated that men make up five to eight percent of all clinical anorectics.

dancers who reported having bulimia versus those reporting anorexia nervosa.

In terms of ethnic/sociocultural influences, white and black female dancers from a number of American regional and national ballet companies were compared. Thirty-three percent of the white American dancers reported having had anorexia and/or bulimia, while none of the black American dancers reported either disorder. The black dancers had more positive body images and were less concerned about dieting than the white dancers, although body weights and hours involved in dance were similar for both groups. The authors postulated that cultural expectations of thinness in the upper-middle-class (the background of most white ballet dancers) might be a significant factor in the development of anorexia, especially when placed in contrast to the perhaps more realistic body images expressed by the black dancers. However, they also point out that the problem may simply be one of reporting; that is, the black dancers in their study may have been less likely to report anorexia if it did not fit in with the expectations of their cultural background.

Level of competition was another important influence on the incidence of eating disorders among dancers. One particularly interesting finding was the fact that even though dancers with national companies had more positive body images and were better adjusted than those with regional companies, there was a higher incidence of eating disorders in the national companies. This finding would seem to contradict the traditional feeling that those dancers with more eating disorders would have more negative body images and exhibit more psychological maladjustment. One possible explanation suggested by the authors is that the highly competitive settings of national companies tend to promote deviant eating behavior because of the rigid standards for weight and body appearance. Eating disorders in these dancers may not be so much a reflection of pre-existing psychological conflicts, but more of the demanding atmospheres in their companies.

The third major factor, genetics, was also intertwined with company demands. Dancers who came from highly selective professional schools tended to exhibit fewer eating disorders than those who had reached professional level via auditions for regional companies. The selected dancers also had a lower incidence of obesity in the family (5 percent) than the nonselected dancers (42 percent). (Incidence of familial obesity in the general population is estimated at 30 percent.) Therefore, the highly-selected dancers in national companies may have a greater genetic predisposition to thinness than their less-selected, regional counterparts. Without genetics on their side, many of the nonselected dancers would have a greater struggle in maintaining the low body weights needed for ballet and might resort to eating-disordered behavior in an effort to achieve or maintain company weight standards.

Hamilton and her colleagues also found that those dancers in national companies who did exhibit problematic eating behavior were heavier than those who did not. The heavier dancers (who were still from 4–10 percent *below* what is considered ideal weight for normal women) consumed fewer calories, exhibited more dieting behavior, and reported more menstrual irregularity than the thinner dancers (who were 11–21 percent below ideal weight for normals). The heavier dancers' diets were also somewhat lower in carbohydrates and significantly lower in iron, niacin, phosphorus, and potassium. Those dancers who also reported they were "terrified of being fat" consumed significantly less protein, fat, iron, and niacin.

As for differences between anorexia and bulimia, while anorectic dancers had different psychological profiles from nonanorectic dancers, there were no overt psychological differences between bulimic and nonbulimic dancers. However, the bulimics did exercise less, had dieted more, and reported that their careers were less important to them than nonbulimics. Previous dieting was the most frequently mentioned reason for binging in this study, although there was no difference in body weight relative to height in bulimics vs. nonbulimics. There was also no difference in body weight between dancers who did and those who did not exhibit anorectic behavior.

While all the studies of Hamilton and her associates were conducted on ballet dancers, Schnitt et al. (1986) looked at a sample of modern dancers to determine the incidence of eating disorders. Although these researchers looked only at anorexia, their subjects did not show anorectic attitudes as frequently as ballet dancers. The study involved 62 high-level, female modern dancers participating in the American Dance Festival. While a small subgroup (8 subjects) did appear to be at risk for anorexia and another 8 were borderline, the majority of the dancers (46 subjects) did not report abnormal eating behavior and were still quite thin (12 percent or more below ideal normal body weight).

There could be several reasons for this difference between ballet and modern dancers. One is that demands for thinness in modern dance are not as extreme as in ballet, and although these modern dancers were nearly as thin as ballet dancers, the professional pressure that one *must* be that thin is perhaps not as great. Another possible influence is the modern dancers' backgrounds. Although the white upper-middle-class origins were similar to the ballet dancers, most of these modern dancers had trained through university departments rather than professional schools. The more broadly-based culture of a university environment might be an important factor in helping dancers avoid problems with eating attitudes. The other possibility is that increased educational opportunities may have allowed these dancers to participate in areas other than dance, so that dance and their weight did not constitute their whole life focus.

The important thing to remember in considering these studies is that they show us that eating disorders are not simply the result of innate psychological or family problems in the dancer. Environmental pressures, cultural background, and genetic, physical endowment appear to play critical roles in determining which dancers are at risk for having an eating disorder. Those involved in setting company and university weight standards may wish to think about these elements in considering how to implement their policies. Dancers who recognize the possibility for an eating disorder within themselves might also wish to consider how they can work towards positive changes in their environment as well as in their own attitudes.

Other Eating Disorders Issues

Because this book promotes increase in activity as a method for controlling weight, it is important that we point out the problem of activity-based anorexia. Researchers Epling and Pierce (1988) feel strongly that a significant number of anorectic cases are the result of "biobehavioral" processes triggered by extensive dieting and exercise. Because strenuous endurance exercise can work to suppress appetite and because the individual who loses weight usually receives positive social feedback, the cycle of food deprivation followed by exercise can reach detrimental levels. These authors base their theory on brain opioids. *Opioids* are neurochemicals that serve to decrease pain and are thought to be responsible for the "runner's high" frequently cited by long-distance runners, and that may relate to the transcendental feelings reported by dancers during training and performance. Therefore, it is theoretically possible to become "addicted" to dieting and exercise. While we hardly mean to imply that by following the advice in this book you will become a weight-loss junkie, keep these feelings in mind.

Another little-known aspect of bulimia is the problem of water intoxication. As we also make a point of suggesting that dancers keep their fluid intake in balance with the physical demands of dance, be aware that water consumption can also go too far. "Binge drinking" has been reported by Salkovskis et al. (1987) in bulimics due to their attempts to cut down on food binges. One subject reported drinking 6 liters of water in a 10-minute period, although measurement of urine output suggested she probably consumed closer to 13 liters. (A liter is about 32 oz.) Because of the rapid changes in sodium levels, which directly affect heart regulation and other critical functions, this type of behavior can be life-threatening. So while it is important for dancers to maintain adequate hydration practices, excessive water consumption on the order of "binge drinking" can be very dangerous.

Treatment for Eating Disorders

Treatment for anorexia nervosa and bulimia have traditionally focused on psychotherapy and cognitive attempts to modify destructive eating behavior. Recently, drug therapies have been introduced which may increase the success rate in dealing with these enigmatic disorders. For anorexia, Drs. Mary Ann Marrazzi and Elliot D. Luby have been studying the effects of a class of drugs known as *opioid inhibitors*. This approach treats anorexia as an addiction to dieting, with drugs such as naltrexone and nalmefene blocking the action of brain opioids and therefore blocking the "dieter's high" we just discussed. Such research, however, is still in the experimental stages.

As for bulimia, anti-depressants appear to offer promising short-term treatment for bulimics, but the long-term success rates are still questionable, with high-relapse rates having been reported after stopping drug therapy. Groups such as Overeaters Anonymous offer a psychological support system patterned after the 12-Step program of Alcoholics Anonymous. At least in the New York area, a number of eating-disorders support groups and counselors are available, but one should pay close attention to credentials and professional affiliations of the staff. Be sure the staff or associates have advanced degrees in psychology, nutrition, and/or medicine. Again, it is important that dancers seek counseling that can address their specific needs.

One of the "real world" problems of securing treatment for eating disorders is payment. Dancers have modest incomes, to say the least, and most insurance companies provide limited coverage, if any, for treatment of eating disorders. If you are involved in directing a university program or professional dance company, the specific language regarding "mental health" benefits in your group's insurance coverage should be carefully reviewed. At a time when health insurance rates are increasing at the same time benefits are decreasing, be sure to read the fine print on your policy to determine if areas where dancers most need coverage are addressed. It is extremely important to consider issues of third-party payment for eating disorders as most reputable programs will otherwise be financially out of reach for dancers. As a company director, discuss this issue with your insurance representative and see if adequate provisions for treatment for eating disorders are included in your policy. As a professional dancer, find out just what your company's health insurance policy covers and what it doesn't. For those involved in a university situation, look into the possibility of help from the psychology, medicine, and/or nutrition departments on your campus.

It is also critically important that any psychological counseling that does take place involve someone who is not just familiar with dancers, but who also understands the dance profession. One psychiatrist writing of his dealings with ballet dancers compared their psychological characteristics to hysterics, obsessives, narcissistics, and schizoids. Such views come from a framework that is not prepared to deal with the unique psychological life of dancers, or any artist for that matter, and can actually result in negative consequences for the dancer. Therefore, it is important to seek counseling from someone who can relate the problems of dancers to the demands of dance. Professional pressures are real and must be dealt with as such. Just because dancers are not *average* (thankfully) does not mean they are not *normal*. And being normal means facing difficult problems that do not necessarily have easy solutions.

Chapter X

Associated Factors Affecting Weight Control

Initial Weight Loss vs. Weight Maintenance

For years it was assumed that *losing* weight was the difficult part of changing one's body composition. Once the weight was lost, the theory went, one could just go back to eating normally and the weight would stay off. But statistics overwhelmingly show that while the majority of dieters do lose weight, it is only the minority that actually keeps it off.

The fact is, losing weight and maintaining the new weight are two separate and distinct entities, as different as sprinting and long-distance running. Failure to appreciate these differences can result in great frustration for the dancer wishing to alter body composition. A recent study examining the results of a weight-loss program immediately after treatment and at one-year follow-up showed some interesting differences in those variables that predicted success (Bonato & Boland, 1987). Factors that contributed to successful weight loss at the end of the 10-week treatment program were measured and compared to factors that contributed to successfully maintaining lost weight at the end of one year.

Those who were most successful in losing weight at the end of the 10-week treatment program had a greater weight loss the first week of the program; set higher monthly weight-loss goals for themselves; and had a greater number of past weight-loss attempts. However, *none* of these factors were important in determining who was successful at maintaining lost weight at one-year follow-up. For those who were successful in maintaining lost weight, there was a greater frequency in being able to overcome urges to overeat; the onset of added weight had occurred at a later age; and there was a greater incidence of employment outside the home than in those who did not maintain their lost weight.

While this study examined obese subjects in a behavioral approach weight-loss program, the important conclusion is that factors affecting initial weight loss and maintenance outcome are not the same. Once a dancer, or anyone for that matter, has achieved his or her initial weight-loss goal, the approach to maintaining lower weight must be specifically considered.

Caloric intake should be slowly and carefully adjusted following attainment of your desired weight. Your exercise schedule should also be gradually adjusted so that you can maintain your new weight. Psychologically, it is important to appreciate that weight modification is not a one-time, temporary program; it involves an ongoing commitment to dietary changes and exercise participation.

Weight Loss and Menstrual Alterations

Many female dancers are used to the "on-again/off-again" relationship they have with their menstrual cycles. In fact, until someone asks them about it, most dancers with irregular periods assume that it's just normal because most of their dance cohorts have similar experiences. The issue of menstrual alterations in relation to dance and weight-loss is one that may not seem to pose an immediate threat to the dancer; however, there are serious short- and long-term consequences related to how menstrual cycles reflect other important bodily functions.

There are three main areas of concern regarding dancers and menstruation: (a) age at which menstruation began, or age at *menarche;* (b) irregular periods or *oligomenorrhea* (missing one to four cycles in a one-year period); and (c) prolonged intervals without menstruating or *amenorrhea* (missing at least five consecutive cycles in a one-year period).

In the late 1970s, researchers in sports medicine began to investigate the prevalence of amenorrhea (lack of periods) in highly-trained female athletes. Typically, these athletes had stopped menstruating when they had entered intense training and would not begin menstruating again until the training had significantly decreased. Initially, physicians and physiologists felt there was little cause for concern because the athletes seemed to go back to having normal cycles and periods once the intense training stopped.

However, as more research emerged, it became clear that prolonged amenorrhea could have significant long-term consequences related to osteoporosis (see Chapter 4). The lack of a menstrual cycle also means that certain female hormones, primarily estrogen, are not being released as they normally would. Estrogen plays a crucial role in the regulation of bone mass, and when estrogen release is diminished, decreased bone density can result.

The effects of prolonged intervals without menstruating have now been well-established by several studies. The most immediate concern to dancers is a known increase in the risk for stress fractures and *scoliosis* (curvature of the spine) in amenorrheic dancers who have stopped menstruating for more than 11-month intervals and/or those who did not start menstruating until age 14 or older (Warren et al., 1986). Benson et al. (1989) have also found an increased incidence of injuries among those dancers with poor nutritional status and menstrual dysfunction. (See also Barrow & Saha, 1988; Cann et al., 1984; Lloyd et al., 1986; Loucks & Horvath, 1985; and Marcus et al., 1985 for similar studies on female athletes.)

This is a particularly difficult area in terms of recommendations because it is also known that certain dancers stop menstruating once they get down to what they consider to be their appropriate dance weight. The Catch-22 appears to be that certain dancers can't seem to both get thin enough to dance professionally and have periods. However, studies have also shown that body weight and body fat alone do not necessarily relate to the dancer's menstrual cycles. Some very thin and lean dancers have periods while others do not. So what is the story here?

One very important factor is the relationship of eating disorders to amenorrhea (Brooks-Gunn et al., 1987). In this study, those dancers who exhibited anorectic or bulimic behavior had a higher incidence of prolonged intervals without menstruation. Although the precise reasons for this are not clear, the nutritional deficits that accompany. eating disorders may be a critical factor.

Another important consideration is our old friend genetics. In terms of age of menarche, genetics does not appear to be the major determining factor (i.e., the age at which your mother started menstruating). Other factors such as intensity of training and eating behavior in the prepubertal years appear to play a greater role in delaying menarche. However, those dancers who are not naturally predisposed to thinness tend to diet more and develop eating disorders more often, which thus puts them at greater risk for having amenorrhea.

So, those are the hard cruel facts. For some dancers, particularly those who are not naturally thin, it appears that getting thin enough for professional ballet standards *may* mean losing their periods, which may then increase their risk for stress fractures and other injuries, as well as scoliosis. Not a pretty picture, but neither is it one that cannot be changed. With eating disorders being an important factor in the development of amenorrhea, there may be a relationship to the deficient nutrient status of the individual. As these studies have shown, having an eating disorder and irregular menses is correlated with *higher* body weights in dancers, rather than lower; so degree of thinness may not be the critical issue in developing menstrual abnormalities.

We must emphasize that no one knows the exact nature of this delicate physiologic balance (some feel that each individual has her own level of "critical fat," below which menstruation ceases), but dancers who go long periods without menstruating, diet regularly, and tend toward extreme eating behavior should try to improve the quality of their food intake as we have previously described, consult a physician for an evaluation of their bone density, and seek professional help regarding their eating behavior.

Premenstrual syndrome and intense cramps upon menstruation can also be problematic for the dancer. Space limits our ability to discuss these topics, so instead we refer you to the following information sources:

National Women's Health Network
1325 G Street NW
Washington, DC 20005
PMS information packet—
$5.00.

American College of Obstetricians and Gynecologists Resource Center
600 Maryland Avenue SW, Suite 300 East
Washington, DC 20024-2588
Brochure "Premenstrual Syndrome" free with self-addressed stamped envelope.

PMS Access
Madison Pharmacy
Associates
Box 9326
Madison, WI 53715
*Information line
800/222-4PMS or
608/833-4PMS in Wisconsin.*

Endometriosis Association
8585 N. 76th Place
Milwaukee, WI 53223
*Information packet on painful
periods and endometriosis.*

Smoking and Caffeine

We won't belabor the health hazards of smoking because we do know that fewer dancers smoke now than ever before. In 1984, Micheli et al. reported that eight out of their nine female ballet subjects smoked, whereas in our 1987 study of 39 ballet and modern dancers, only seven were smokers (Chmelar et al.). The greatest concern about quitting among dancers who smoke is the prospect of gaining weight. In fact, among university women who smoke, nearly 40 percent use it as a dietary strategy (Klesges & Klesges, 1988). Of those who quit smoking only to start again, 36 percent report weight gain and increased appetite as reasons for the relapse. However, we encourage you to carefully consider the sections in this book on cardiovascular endurance and weight loss relative to smoking. Smoking will diminish your aerobic capacity and therefore interfere with exercise aimed at weight loss.

We will also bring up one rarely mentioned point about cigarettes: American cigarettes tend to contain a lot of sugar, which some researchers believe increases the risk of lung cancer (Passey et al., 1966). Smokers also tend to consume more sugar in their diets than nonsmokers (Bennett et al., 1970); however, it is not known if the dietary consumption of sugar is related to the development of cancer.

Caffeine consumption is another habit which gets mixed up in the fear of weight gain. Not only can caffeine stimulate appetite by causing decreases in blood glucose levels, but caffeine is extremely detrimental in terms of calcium absorption. As previously mentioned, a high caffeine intake is one of the risk factors associated with osteoporosis. (An intake of 200 mg/day of caffeine is considered moderate.) We certainly don't intend to preach on the hazards of any and all chemicals, but if you are getting more than 250 mg of caffeine a day, consider the benefits of cutting down. The average caffeine content of various products is listed in Table 10.1.

Fads and Frauds

Just when you think every diet or supplement fad that could ever possibly grace the pages of publishing has finally sailed into oblivion, some new "fat magnet" comes along to take consumers' money, time, and hopes. We have tried to emphasize the physiologic rationale behind our recommendations, and to drive home the point that there is no magic supplement for losing weight. Nevertheless, we know the claims for super weight-loss formulas and "fat melting" pills become awfully enticing when you're trudging through 45 minutes of aerobic exercise and looking forward to a dinner of skinless turkey, potato, and green beans.

Table 10.1: Average Caffeine Content of Various Products

Beverages/Food*	Serving Size	Caffeine (mg)
Coffee, brewed (drip)†	5 oz	115
Coffee, instant	5 oz (1 tsp)	65
Coffee, decaffeinated	5 oz	3
Tea, brewed, U.S. brands	5 oz	40
Tea, brewed, imported brands	5 oz	60
Tea, iced	12 oz	70
Coca-Cola (regular & diet)	12 oz	46
Pepsi-Cola (regular & diet)	12 oz	36
Mountain Dew	12 oz	59
Cocoa	5 oz	4
Milk chocolate	1 oz	6
Dark chocolate (semi-sweet)	1 oz	20

Nonprescription Drugs*	Standard Dose	Caffeine (mg)
Anacin	2	64
Excedrin	2	130
Aqua-Ban (diuretic)	1	100
Appetite control aids *(Dietac, Dexatrim, Codexin)*	1	200

*Read labels carefully to determine if a product not listed contains caffeine.
†Caffeine content varies for coffee and tea depending on type of bean or tea leaf, as well as method of beverage preparation. These values are based on averages.
Source: *FDA Consumer*, March 1984, Food and Drug Administration.

Because of the high value they place on keeping their bodies perfectly tuned, dancers are particularly vulnerable when it comes to claims for vitamin and mineral "super" formulas. Before investing any money into such supplements, be sure to read the article "Foods, Drugs, or Frauds?" in the May 1985 issue of *Consumer Reports* (your local or campus library should have a copy). The article provides a chilling account of the claims and actual contents of various nutrition supplements. Just to give you a flavor of what was contained in the article, consider the following lab analysis of five ounces of a popular supplement known as Blue Green Manna: "15 whole or equivalent adult flies, 164 adult fly fragments, 41 whole or equivalent maggots, 59 maggot fragments, one ant, five ant fragments, one adult cicada, one cicada pupa, 763 insect fragments, nine ticks, four mites, 1000 ostracods, two rat or mouse hairs, four bird feathers, six bird-feather barbules, and 10,500 water fleas." Fortunately, the FDA seized Blue Green Manna products in 1983 as unsafe food additives.

The point is that herbal supplements, vitamins, and minerals come under a grey area in terms of FDA regulation, and with so many other problems to combat, the FDA is underequipped to deal with the flood of potentially unsafe nutritional supplements. Don't assume that vitamins and minerals are packaged in non-toxic doses: this can and does happen. Let the dancer beware and pay particular attention to the kind of supplements you consume. Be extra careful with mail-order supplements and those distributed through individuals on a "club" basis.

This is not to say you should avoid appropriate vitamin and mineral supplementation, but substances such as "kidney extract," "raw prostrate," and "raw bovine stomach tissue concentrate" (yes, these are actual products) can be potentially harmful. Oral chelation supplements, which are often touted as being superior, are actually no more than overly potent, overly expensive vitamins and should be used with caution due to the potential for overdose of such toxic vitamins as A and D. Another temptation for dancers, herbal weight-loss formulas, are often nothing more than laxatives.

In exercise physiology, there is a whole subset of study devoted to what are known as "ergogenic aids," which simply means any substance that enhances performance. These "work" aids range from vitamins to steroids and from benign to life-threatening. So far, no substance has been found to actually improve performance without the risk of harmful side-effects. However, there are many nutritional supplements that elicit no performance enhancement under conditions of formal study, but yet have many users who swear by their beneficial effects.

In short, we fully realize that there are elements of performance that no scientist can measure and that if you have found a particular combination of *safe* supplements that seems to positively affect your dancing, then perhaps it is. On the other hand, be aware that your first approach should entail improving your basic nutritional status. Experimentation beyond that is up to you, just be particularly careful about overdoses of fat-soluble vitamins and overdoses of money to someone making golden promises.

Towards a Better, Healthier Dancer

We set out to accomplish two things in this book: (a) to provide diet and exercise information to dancers that would help them achieve their weight modification goals, and (b) to provide nutritional information that would help dancers improve the quality of their diets. In the context of these issues, we hope we have shed some light on why it is so difficult for some dancers to maintain their weight and not others; on how the physical and psychological elements of the body interact; and on how to set realistic goals in terms of balancing health and career goals.

We also hope that some of the information we have presented concerning genetics and body type will not be discouraging to those of you who find yourselves having to consider whether or not your genetic endowment is suited to a particular style of dance. The dancer discussed in the introduction, who went from overweight dance student to top professional by changing her dietary and exercise habits, also went from ballet to modern dance. She found herself not only better suited for modern dance physically, but mentally as well. This is not to say everyone whose weight is a problem should consider changing styles, but rather, the important thing is to find the medium in which you can best express yourself.

Fortunately for all of us, dance is never static. It is a constantly changing form that encompasses performances ranging from the classics of New York City Ballet to the carnation-covered stages of Pina Bausch, and from the spectacular productions of "Cats" to the intimate performances of Ann Carlson. So, wherever your special contribution to dance establishes itself, we hope the information in this book will help you improve both your performance capabilities and your health via better diet and nutrition.

Appendix A **Exchange Lists**

These exchange lists are reprinted with the permission of the American Diabetes Association and American Dietetic Association, who state:

"The exchange lists are the basis of a meal planning system designed by a committee of the American Diabetes Association and The American Dietetic Association. While designed primarily for people with diabetes and others who must follow special diets, the exchange lists are based on principles of good nutrition that apply to everyone. © 1986 American Diabetes Association, The American Dietetic Association."

1. Starch/Bread List

Each item in this list contains approximately 15 grams of carbohydrate, 3 grams of protein, a trace of fat, and 80 calories. Whole grain products average about 2 grams of fiber per serving. Those foods that contain 3 or more grams of fiber per serving are identified with the symbol *.

CEREALS/GRAINS/PASTA
(Count as 1 starch exchange)

*Bran cereals, concentrated (i.e., Bran Buds®, All Bran®)	⅓ cup
*Bran cereals, flaked	½ cup
Bulgur (cooked)	½ cup
Cooked cereals	½ cup
Cornmeal (dry)	2½ Tbsp.
Grapenuts	3 Tbsp.
Grits (cooked)	½ cup
Other ready-to-eat unsweetened cereals	¾ cup
Pasta (cooked)	½ cup
Puffed cereal	½ cup
Rice, white or brown (cooked)	⅓ cup
Shredded wheat	½ cup
*Wheat germ	3 Tbsp.

DRIED BEANS/PEAS/LENTILS

*Beans and peas (cooked) (i.e., kidney, white, split, blackeye)	⅓ cup
*Lentils (cooked)	⅓ cup
*Baked beans	¼ cup

STARCHY VEGETABLES

*Corn	½ cup
*Corn on cob, 6 in. long	1
*Lima beans	½ cup
*Peas, green (canned or frozen)	½ cup
*Plantain	½ cup
Potato, baked	1 small (3 oz)
Potato, mashed	½ cup
Squash, winter (acorn, butternut)	¾ cup
Yam, sweet potato, plain	⅓ cup

BREAD

Bagel	½ (1 oz)
Bread sticks, crisp, 4 in. long x ½ in.	2 (⅔ oz)
Croutons, low fat	1 cup
English muffin	½

Frankfurter or hamburger bun	½ (1 oz)
Pita, 6 in. across	½
Plain roll, small	1 (1 oz)
Raisin bread, unfrosted	1 slice (1 oz)
*Rye, pumpernickel	1 slice (1 oz)
Tortilla, 6 in. across	1
White bread (including French and Italian)	1 slice (1 oz)
Whole wheat bread	1 slice (1 oz)

CRACKERS/SNACKS

Animal crackers	8
Graham crackers, 2½ in. square	3
Matzoth	¾ oz
Melba toast	5 slices
Oyster crackers	24
Popcorn (popped, no fat added)	3 cups
Pretzels	¾ oz
Rye crisp, 2 in. x 3½ in.	4
Saltine-type crackers	6

Whole wheat crackers, no fat added (i.e., Finn®, Kavli®, Wasa®)	2–4 slices (¾ oz)

STARCH FOODS PREPARED WITH FAT

(Count as 1 STARCH exchange plus 1 FAT exchange)

Biscuit, 2½ in. across	1
Chow mein noodles	½ cup
Corn bread, 2 in. cube	1 (2 oz)
Cracker, round butter type	6
French fried potatoes, 2 in. to 3½ in. long	10 (1½ oz)
Muffin, plain, small	1
Pancake, 4 in. across	2
Stuffing, bread (prepared)	¼ cup
Taco shell, 6 in. across	2
Waffle, 4½ in. square	1
Whole wheat crackers, fat added (i.e., Triscuits®)	4–6 (1 oz)

2. Meat List

Each serving of meat and substitutes on this list contains about 7 grams of protein. The amount of fat and number of calories varies, depending on what kind of meat or substitute you choose.

The list is divided into three parts: LEAN MEAT, MEDIUM-FAT MEAT, and HIGH-FAT MEAT. One meat exchange, one ounce after cooking, of each of these includes:

	Carbo-hydrate (grams)	Protein (grams)	Fat (grams)	Calories
LEAN MEAT	0	7	3	55
MEDIUM-FAT MEAT	0	7	5	75
HIGH-FAT MEAT	0	7	8	100

LEAN MEAT AND SUBSTITUTES

(One exchange is equal to any one of the following items)
Meats and substitutes that have 400 mg or more of sodium per exchange are marked with the symbol §.

Beef: USDA Good or Choice grades of lean beef, such as round, sirloin, and flank steak; tenderloin; and chipped beef(§)   1 oz

Pork: Lean pork, such as fresh ham; canned, cured or boiled ham(§); Canadian bacon, tenderloin. — 1 oz

Veal: All cuts are lean except for veal cutlets (ground or cubed). Examples are lean veal chops and roasts. — 1 oz

Poultry: Chicken, turkey, Cornish hen (without skin) — 1 oz

Fish: All fresh and frozen fish — 1 oz

Crab, lobster, scallops, shrimp, clams(§) (fresh or canned in water) — 2 oz

Oysters — 6 med

Tuna(§) (canned in water) — ¼ cup

Herring (uncreamed or smoked) — 1 oz

Sardines (canned) — 2 med

Wild Game: Venison, rabbit, squirrel — 1 oz

Pheasant, duck, goose (without skin) — 1 oz

Cheese: Any cottage cheese — ¼ cup

Grated parmesan — 2 Tbsp

Diet cheeses(§) (less than 55 calories per oz) — 1 oz

Other: 95% fat-free luncheon meat — 1 oz

Egg whites — 3 whites

Egg substitutes (less than 55 calories per ¼ cup) — ¼ cup

HIGH-FAT MEAT AND SUBSTITUTES
(We count HIGH-FAT MEATS in our dietary guidelines as a combination LEAN MEAT and FAT)

Beef: Most USDA Prime cuts of beef, such as ribs, corned beef(§) — 1 oz

Pork: Spareribs, ground pork, pork sausage(§) (patty or link) — 1 oz

Lamb: Patties (ground lamb) — 1 oz

Fish: Any fried fish product — 1 oz

Cheese: All regular cheeses(§), i.e., American, Blue, Cheddar, Monterey, Swiss — 1 oz

Other: Luncheon meat(§), i.e., bologna, salami, pimento loaf — 1 oz

Sausage(§), i.e., Polish, Italian — 1 oz

Knockwurst, smoked — 1 oz

Bratwurst(§) — 1 oz

Frankfurter(§) (turkey or chicken) — 1 frank (10/lb)

Peanut butter (contains unsaturated fat) — 1 Tbsp

Count as one high-fat meat plus one fat exchange: Frankfurter(§) (beef, pork, or combination) — 1 frank (10/lb)

MEDIUM-FAT MEAT AND SUBSTITUTES
(We count MEDIUM-FAT MEATS in our dietary guidelines as a combination LEAN MEAT and FAT)

Beef: Most beef products. Examples are: all ground beef, roast (rib, chuck, rump), steak (cubed, Porterhouse, T-bone), and meatloaf — 1 oz

Pork: Most pork products. Examples are: chops, loin roast, Boston butt, cutlets — 1 oz

Lamb: Most lamb products. Examples are: chops, leg, roast — 1 oz

Veal: Cutlet (ground or cubed, unbreaded) — 1 oz

Fish: Tuna(§) (canned in oil and drained) — ¼ cup

Salmon(§) (canned) — ¼ cup

Cheese: All regular cheeses(§), i.e., American, Blue, Cheddar, Monterey, Swiss	1 oz
Other: 86% fat-free luncheon meat(§)	1 oz

Egg (high in cholesterol, limit to 3 per week)	1
Egg substitutes with 56–80 calories per ¼ cup	¼ cup
Tofu (2½ in. × 2¾ in. × 1 in.)	4 oz
Liver, heart, kidney, sweetbreads (high cholesterol)	1 oz

3. Vegetable List

Each vegetable exchange contains about 5 grams of carbohydrate, 2 grams of protein, and 25 calories. Vegetables contain 2–3 grams of dietary fiber. Vegetables which contain more than 400 mg of sodium per serving are marked with the symbol (§). Unless otherwise noted, one vegetable exchange is:

½ cup of cooked vegetables or vegetable juice
1 cup of raw vegetables

Artichoke (½ medium)	Mushrooms, Cooked
Asparagus	Okra
Beans (green, wax, Italian)	Onion
Bean sprouts	Pea pods

Beets	Peppers (green)
Broccoli	Rutabaga
Brussels sprouts	Sauerkraut(§)
Cabbage, cooked	Spinach
Carrots	Summer Squash
Cauliflower	Tomato (one large)
Eggplant	Tomato/ vegetable juice(§)
Greens (collard, mustard, turnip)	Turnips
Kohlrabi	Water chestnuts
Leeks	Zucchini, cooked

Starchy vegetables such as corn, peas, and potatoes are found on the STARCH/ BREAD list. For free vegetables, see FREE FOOD LIST.

4. Fruit List

Each item on this list contains about 15 grams of carbohydrate and 60 calories. Fresh, frozen, and dry fruits have about 2 grams of fiber per serving. Fruits that have 3 or more grams of fiber per serving are marked with the symbol *. The carbohydrate and caloric content for a fruit serving are based on the usual serving of the most commonly eaten fruits. Use fresh fruits or fruits frozen or canned without sugar added. Unless otherwise noted, the serving size for one fruit exchange is:

½ cup of fresh fruit or fruit juice
¼ cup dried fruit

FRESH, FROZEN, AND UNSWEETENED CANNED FRUIT

Apple (raw, 2 in. across)	1 apple
Applesauce (unsweetened)	½ cup
Apricots (medium, raw)	4 apricots
Apricots (canned)	½ cup, or 4 halves
Banana (9 in. long)	½ banana
*Blackberries (raw)	¾ cup
*Blueberries (raw)	¾ cup
Cantaloupe (5 in. across)	⅓ melon
Cantaloupe cubes	1 cup
Cherries (large, raw)	12 cherries

Cherries (canned)	½ cup
Figs (raw, 2 in. across)	2 figs
Fruit cocktail (canned)	½ cup
Grapefruit (medium)	½ grapefruit
Grapefruit (segments)	¾ cup
Grapes (small)	15 grapes
Honeydew melon (medium)	⅛ melon
Honeydew melon, cubes	1 cup
Kiwi (large)	1 kiwi
Mandarin oranges	¾ cup
Mango (small)	½ mango
*Nectarine (1½ in. across)	1 nectarine
Orange (2½ in. across)	1 orange
Papaya	1 cup
Peach (2¾ in. across)	1 peach
Peach, slices	¾ cup
Peaches (canned)	½ cup, or 2 halves
Pear	½ large, or 1 small
Pears (canned)	½ cup, or 2 halves
Persimmon (medium, native)	2 persimmons
Pineapple (raw)	¾ cup
Pineapple (canned)	⅓ cup
Plum (raw, 2 in. across)	2 plums
*Pomegranate	1 cup
*Raspberries (raw)	1 cup
*Strawberries (raw, Whole)	1¼ cup
Tangerine (2½ in. across)	2 tangerines
Watermelon (cubes)	1¼ cup

DRIED FRUIT

*Apples	4 rings
*Apricots	7 halves
Dates	2½ medium
*Figs	1½
*Prunes	3 medium
Raisins	2 Tbsp

FRUIT JUICE

Apple juice/cider	½ cup
Cranberry juice cocktail	⅓ cup
Grapefruit	½ cup
Grape juice	⅓ cup
Orange juice	½ cup
Pineapple juice	½ cup
Prune juice	⅓ cup

5. Milk List

Each serving of milk or milk products on this list contains about 12 grams of carbohydrate and 8 grams of protein. The amount of fat in milk is measured in percent (%) of butterfat. The list is divided into three parts based on the amount of fat and calories: SKIM MILK, LOWFAT MILK, and WHOLE MILK. One exchange of each of these includes:

	Carbohydrate (grams)	Protein (grams)	Fat (grams)	Calories
SKIM/VERY LOWFAT	12	8	trace	90
LOWFAT	12	8	5	120
WHOLE	12	8	8	150

SKIM AND VERY LOWFAT MILK

(Our dietary guidelines are based on Skim Milk products)

Skim milk	1 cup
½% milk	1 cup
1% milk	1 cup
Lowfat buttermilk	1 cup
Evaporated skim milk	½ cup

| Dry nonfat milk | ⅓ cup |
| Plain nonfat yogurt | 8 oz |

LOWFAT MILK

| 2% milk | 1 cup |
| Plain lowfat yogurt (with added nonfat milk solids) | 8 oz |

WHOLE MILK (3¼% butterfat)
(We do not include Whole Milk in our dietary guidelines)

Whole milk	1 cup
Evaporated whole milk	½ cup
Whole plain yogurt	8 oz

6. Fat List

Each serving on the FAT list contains 5 grams of fat, and 45 calories. The foods on the fat list contain mostly fat, although some may also contain a small amount of protein. All fats are high in calories and should be carefully measured. Fats that have more than 400 mg of sodium per *two* servings are marked with†.

UNSATURATED FATS

Avocado	⅛ medium
Margarine	1 tsp
†Margarine, diet	1 Tbsp
Mayonnaise	1 tsp
†Mayonnaise, reduced-calorie	1 Tbsp
Nuts and Seeds:	
Almonds, dry roasted	6 whole
Cashews, dry roasted	1 Tbsp
Pecans	2 whole
Peanuts	20 small or 10 large
Walnuts	2 whole
Other nuts	1 Tbsp
Seeds, pine nuts, sunflower	1 Tbsp
Pumpkin seeds	2 tsp

Oil (corn, cottonseed, safflower, soybean, sunflower, olive, peanut)	1 tsp
†Olives	10 small or 5 large
Salad dressing, mayonnaise-type	2 tsp
Salad dressing, mayonnaise-type, reduced-calorie	1 Tbsp
†Salad dressing (all varieties)	1 Tbsp
Salad dressing, reduced-calorie(§)	2 Tbsp

SATURATED FATS

Butter	1 tsp
†Bacon	1 slice
Chitterlings	½ oz
Coconut, shredded	2 Tbsp
Coffee whitener, liquid	2 Tbsp
Coffee whitener, powder	4 tsp
Cream (light, coffee, table)	2 Tbsp
Cream, sour	2 Tbsp
Cream (heavy, whipping)	1 Tbsp
Cream cheese	1 Tbsp
†Salt pork	¼ oz

Free Foods

A free food is any food or drink that contains less than 20 calories per serving.

DRINKS

Bouillon(§) or broth without fat
Bouillon, low-sodium
Carbonated drinks, sugar-free
Carbonated water
Club soda
Cocoa powder, unsweetened (1 Tbsp)
Coffee/Tea
Drink mixes, sugar-free
Tonic water, sugar-free

FRUIT
Cranberries,
  unsweetened,
  ½ cup
Rhubarb,
  unsweetened,
  ½ cup

**NONSTICK PAN
SPRAY**

SALAD GREENS
Endive
Escarole
Lettuce
Romaine
Spinach

VEGETABLES
  (raw, 1 cup)
Cabbage

Celery
Chinese
  cabbage*
Cucumber
Green onion
Hot peppers
Mushrooms
Radishes
Zucchini*

**SWEET
SUBSTITUTES**
Candy, hard,
  sugar-free
Gelatin, sugar-
  free
Gum, sugar-free

CONDIMENTS
Catsup
Horseradish

Mustard
Pickles(§), dill,
  unsweetened
Salad dressing,
  low-calorie,
  2 Tbsp
Taco sauce,
  1 Tbsp
Vinegar

Jam/Jelly, sugar-
  free 2 tsp
Pancake syrup,
  sugar-free 1–2
  Tbsp
Sugar substitutes
  (saccharin,
  aspartame)
Whipped topping,
  2 Tbsp

SEASONINGS
Herbs, spices, flavoring extracts, lemon or lime juice, garlic, soy sauce, and Worcestershire sauce may be used without restriction; however, be careful of the sodium content in some condiments.

Nutritional Content and Exchanges for Frozen Dinners Under 300 Calories

Brand name items are used to demonstrate how to calculate exchanges according to caloric, protein, fat, and carbohydrate content; however, we are not recommending one brand over another, nor are we recommending premade dinners in lieu of home cooked meals. Rather, we recognize that many dancers prefer to purchase such dinners, and therefore we use them here and in Appendices C and D as examples of the type of item that you might purchase and how they fit into a diet using the Exchange System.

Brand and Type	Calories	Protein (g)	Carb (g)	Fat (g)	Sodium (mg)
Armour Dinner Classic Lite					
Chicken Oriental	230	23	30	2	920
Exchanges:	MEAT*: 3.0, STARCH: 1.5, VEG: 1.0, *Omit* 2 FAT				
Budget Gourmet Slim Selects					
Chicken Au Gratin	260	19	21	11	960
Exchanges:	MEAT: 2.5, STARCH: 1.0, FAT: 0.5, VEG: 1.0				
French Recipe Chicken	260	20	22	10	970
Exchanges:	MEAT: 2.5, STARCH: 1.0, FAT: 0.5, VEG: 1.0				
Glazed Turkey	270	17	39	5	760
Exchanges:	MEAT: 2.0, STARCH: 2.0, FAT: 0.0, VEG: 1.0				
Linguini/Scallops/ Clams	280	16	28	11	630
Exchanges:	MEAT: 2.0, STARCH: 1.5, FAT: 1.0, VEG: 1.0				
Oriental Beef	290	17	36	9	810
Exchanges:	MEAT: 2.0, STARCH: 2.0, FAT: 0.5, VEG: 0.5				
Sirloin Beef/Herb Sauce	290	19	27	12	770
Exchanges:	MEAT: 2.5, STARCH: 1.5, FAT: 0.5, VEG: 1.0				
Celentano					
Broccoli Stuffed Shells	231	10	14	15	360
Exchanges:	MEAT: 1.0, STARCH: 1.0, FAT: 2.0, VEG: 1.0				

Brand and Type	Calories	Protein (g)	Carb (g)	Fat (g)	Sodium (mg)
Lasagna Primavera	300	17	36	9	500
Exchanges:	MEAT: 2.0, STARCH: 2.0, FAT: 0.5, VEG: 1.0				
Manicotti	300	18	22	15	435
Exchanges:	MEAT: 2.0, STARCH: 1.5, FAT: 2.0, VEG: 0.0				
Healthy Choice					
Oriental Pepper Steak	290	23	35	6	510
Exchanges:	MEAT: 2.5, STARCH: 1.0, VEG: 1.0, FRUIT: 1.0				
Shrimp Creole	210	8	42	1	560
Exchanges:	MEAT: 0.5, STARCH: 1.5, VEG: 1.0, FRUIT: 1.0				
Sweet & Sour Chicken	280	22	44	2	260
Exchanges:	MEAT: 2.0, STARCH: 1.0, VEG: 1.0, FRUIT: 1.0				
Lean Cuisine (Stouffer's)					
Chicken Cacciatore	280	23	25	10	950
Exchanges:	MEAT: 2.5, STARCH: 1.0, FAT: 0.5, VEG: 2.0				
Glazed Chicken	270	26	23	5	710
Exchanges:	MEAT: 3.0, STARCH: 1.0, FAT: 0.0, VEG: 0.0				
Linguini/Clam Sauce	260	16	32	7	800
Exchanges:	MEAT: 1.5, STARCH: 2.0, FAT: 0.5, VEG: 0.5				
Zucchini Lasagna	260	21	28	7	975
Exchanges:	MEAT: 2.0, STARCH: 1.5, FAT: 0.0, VEG: 1.0				
Le Menu (Swanson)					
Sliced Turkey Breast	270	17	37	6	1,020
Exchanges:	MEAT: 1.5, STARCH: 2.5, FAT: 0.0, VEG: 0.5				
Le Menu Light					
Stuffed Cheese Shells	280	16	35	8	720
Exchanges:	MEAT: 1.5, STARCH: 2.0, FAT: 0.5, VEG: 1.5				
Mrs. Paul's Light Entrée					
Fish Au Gratin	280	35	14	9	1,100
Exchanges:	MEAT: 4.5, STARCH: 1.0, *Omit* 1 FAT				
Seafood Rotini	280	14	40	7	720
Exchanges:	MEAT: 1.5, STARCH: 2.0, FAT: 0.0, VEG: 2.0				
Swanson Homestyle Dinners					
Sirloin Tips	270	17	27	10	570
Exchanges:	MEAT: 2.0, STARCH: 1.5, FAT: 1.0, VEG: 0.5				
Veal Parmesan	280	14	22	15	880
Exchanges:	MEAT: 1.5, STARCH: 1.5, FAT: 2.0, VEG: 0.0				
Tyson Gourmet Selections					
Chicken Marsala	300	19	26	13	900
Exchanges:	MEAT: 2.0 STARCH: 1.5, FAT: 2.0, VEG: 0.5				

Brand and Type	Calories	Protein (g)	Carb (g)	Fat (g)	Sodium (g)
Weight Watchers†					
Imperial Chicken	230	22	26	4	950
Exchanges:	MEAT: 2.0, STARCH: 1.5, FAT: 0.0, VEG: 1.0				
Sweet and Sour Chicken	250	15	42	2	590
Exchanges:	MEAT: 1.0, STARCH: 2.0, FAT: 0.0, VEG: 2.0				

*MEAT = LEAN MEAT

†Note: Exchanges listed on *Weight Watchers* products are different from the exchanges we list. Our exchanges are based on the American Diabetic Association Exchange Lists, whereas *Weight Watchers* has their own exchange system.

Appendix C Exchanges for "Goodie" Foods

Item	Amount	Exchanges	Approximate Total Calories
Ice Cream			
Breyer's			
Cookies & Cream	½ cup	1 FRUIT, 2 FAT, ½ MILK	170
Vanilla "Light"	½ cup	½ FRUIT, 1 FAT, ½ MILK	120
Häagen Dazs			
Vanilla	½ cup	1½ FRUIT, 3 FAT, ½ MILK	260
Deep Chocolate	½ cup	2 FRUIT, 3 FAT, ½ MILK	290
Sorbet & Cream:	½ cup	1½ FRUIT, 1½ FAT, ½ MILK	190
Lime, Blueberry			
Sealtest			
Vanilla	½ cup	1 FRUIT, 1½ FAT, ½ MILK	140
Frozen Yogurt			
Yoplait Vanilla	½ cup	½ FRUIT, 1 FAT, ½ MILK	125
Élan Chocolate	½ cup	1 FRUIT, ½ FAT, ½ MILK	130
Ice Milk			
Steve's Gourmet Light			
Cookies & Cream	½ cup	1 FRUIT, 1 FAT, 1 MILK	200
Vanilla	½ cup	1 FRUIT, 1 FAT, 1 MILK	190
Weight Watchers	½ cup	½ FRUIT, ½ FAT, ½ MILK	100
Swiss Vanilla			
Non-Dairy Frozen Dessert			
Tofutti Chocolate	½ cup	1 STARCH, 2 FAT, ½ FRUIT	210
Supreme			
Sherbet			
Sealtest, All flavors	½ cup	1 FRUIT, 1 STARCH	140
Cookies:			
Nabisco			
Oreos, Chips Ahoy	2	½ STARCH, 1 FAT	90
Fig Newtons	2	1 STARCH, ½ FRUIT	100
Pepperidge Farm			
Bordeaux	3	1 STARCH, 1 FAT	110
Milano	3	1 STARCH, 2 FAT	180
Orange Milano	3	1½ STARCH, 3 FAT	230
Milk Chocolate	3	1 STARCH, 3 FAT	210
Macademia			
Frookie Oat Bran	3	½ STARCH, 1 FRUIT, 1 FAT	135

Item	Amount	Exchanges	Approximate Total Calories
Beer/4.5% alcohol*	12 oz	1 STARCH, 2 FAT	150
Bud Natural Light	12 oz	1 STARCH, 1½ FAT	110
Schlitz Light	12 oz	½ STARCH, 1 fat	95
Table wine/12% alcohol	3 oz	½ FRUIT, 1 FAT	75
"Hard" liquor Vodka, Rum, Scotch	1½ oz	3 FAT	125
Liqueurs Amaretto, Anisette, Kahlua	1 oz	½ FRUIT, 1 FAT	85
Popcorn (popped) *Orville Redenbacher's Microwave Natural†*	3 cups	½ STARCH, 1 FAT	80
Orville Redenbacher's Microwave Light Butter	3 cups	1 STARCH	50
Pop Secret Natural	3 cups	1 STARCH, 1½ FAT	140
Pop Secret Light	3 cups	½ STARCH, 1 FAT	90
Brie, Camembert Cheese	1 oz	1 LEAN MEAT, 1 FAT	90
Feta Cheese	1 oz	½ LEAN MEAT, 1 FAT	75
Pizza, cheese, regular crust	¼ of 10 in. pie	2 STARCH, 1 LEAN MEAT, 2 FAT	280

*Most alcoholic beverages contain no actual fat; however, the alcohol is accounted for under the FAT category because of its caloric density.

†Different brands of microwave popcorn vary in their caloric and fat content.

Menus for Meal Planning

The following menus are intended to help you design your own daily diet plans. Each menu is calculated to provide approximately 60 percent of calories from carbohydrate, 20 percent from protein, and 20 percent from fat. These are *low-fat* diets intended to help promote weight loss. For a healthy maintenance diet, fat may be increased to 30 percent, with carbohydrate and protein each decreased between 5 and 10 percent. Foods are grouped according to the Exchange System, which was detailed in Appendix A. Some foods must be accounted for by combinations of exchanges. Caloric and gram values are approximate, and remember, you can also include "free" foods of your choice.

These food selections focus on the areas in which dancers tend to be deficient, i.e., B_6, folic acid, B_{12}, pantothenic acid, biotin, iron, calcium, magnesium, and zinc. Basic meal and snack plans can be added to or subtracted from to fit a higher or lower caloric intake.

We have started our diets at 1,000 kcal/day, which may seem high to those dancers who are used to 600 kcal diets. However, remember that these diets are *low-fat* and are designed to be used in conjunction with the aerobic exercise plan outlined earlier. We suggest that for overall health and nutritional reasons, you try to go no lower than 1,000 kcal/day in your weight control efforts.

Menu for 1,000 kcal/day Diet: #1

Breakfast
¾ cup *Cheerios* cereal	1 STARCH
½ cup skim milk	½ SKIM MILK
½ banana	1 FRUIT
Decaf coffee or tea	

Snack
½ medium-large apple	1 FRUIT

Lunch
¼ cup canned in water tuna	1 LEAN MEAT
Mix to make 2 cups: raw mushrooms, broccoli, beets	2 VEGETABLE
1 tsp olive oil, plus vinegar or lemon juice to taste	1 FAT
1 slice whole wheat bread	1 STARCH

Snack
½ cup vegetable juice cocktail	1 VEGETABLE

1 cup plain nonfat yogurt	1 SKIM MILK
½ slice whole wheat bread	½ STARCH
1 Tbsp peanut butter/ricotta cheese spread*	½ LEAN MEAT, ½ FAT

Dinner

| 1½ oz skinless turkey breast | 1 LEAN MEAT |
| 1½ cup salad: tomato, artichoke hearts (canned in water), Romaine lettuce | 1 VEGETABLE |

½ cup cooked carrot	1 VEGETABLE
1 Tbsp 1000 Island dressing made with "Light" mayonnaise	1 FAT
1 small baked potato	1 STARCH
½ cup strawberries with	½ FRUIT
½ cup low-fat vanilla yogurt	½ FAT, ½ SKIM MILK

*To make: mix ¼ cup natural peanut butter, 1 cup low-fat ricotta chese, ½ tsp cinnamon, 1 tsp vanilla extract.

Exchange Totals for 1,000 kcal/day Diet: #1

	STARCH	LEAN MEAT	VEG	FRUIT	SKIM MILK	FAT	Total
EXCH	3.5	2.5	5	2.5	2	3	
Carb (g)	52.5	0	25	37.5	24	0	139.0
Pro (g)	12	17.5	10	0	16	0	55.5
Fat (g)	0	7.5	0	0	tr	15	22.5
Kcal	280	137.5	125	150	180	135	1,007.5

Menu for 1,200 kcal/day Diet: #2

Breakfast

¼ cup quick-cooking oats, *uncooked*	1 STARCH
1 cup non-fat plain yogurt	1 SKIM MILK
3 medium prunes, sliced	1 FRUIT
1 chopped walnut (Mix oats, yogurt, prunes, nuts)	½ FAT

Snack

| 1 cup tomato juice | 2 VEGETABLE |
| ½ oz Jack cheese | ½ FAT, ½ LEAN MEAT |

Lunch

3 low-salt, low-fat crackers	½ STARCH
½ oz 95% fat-free ham	½ LEAN MEAT
½ Tbsp "light" mayonnaise Mustard to taste	½ FAT

1 slice whole wheat bread	1 STARCH
1 cup raw broccoli/ zucchini	1 VEGETABLE

Snack

1 cup skim milk	1 SKIM MILK
½ banana	1 FRUIT

Dinner

Budget Gourmet Slim Select Glazed Turkey	2 LEAN MEAT, 2 STARCH, 1 VEGETABLE

1½ cup fresh spinach, tomato	1 VEGETABLE
1 tsp olive oil, ½ tsp vinegar	1 FAT
½ cup *Breyer's* "Light" vanilla ice cream	½ SKIM MILK, ½ FRUIT, 1 FAT
1/3 cup blueberries	½ FRUIT

Exchange Totals for 1,200 kcal/day Diet: #2

	STARCH	LEAN MEAT	VEG	FRUIT	SKIM MILK	FAT	Total
EXCH	4.5	3	5	3	2.5	3.5	
Carb (g)	67.5	0	25	45	30	0	167.5 g
Pro (g)	13.5	21	10	0	20	0	64.5 g
Fat (g)	0	9	0	0	tr	17.5	26.5 g
Kcal	360	165	125	180	225	157.5	1,212.5 kcal

Menu for 1,350 kcal/day Diet: #3

Breakfast

1 slice whole wheat toast	1 STARCH
1 tsp margarine	1 FAT
2 Tbsp scrambled egg substitute	½ LEAN MEAT
½ cup skim milk	½ SKIM MILK
½ cup orange juice	1 FRUIT

Snack

½ banana	1 FRUIT
1 Tbsp cream cheese	1 FAT
½ bagel	1 STARCH

Lunch

Lean Cuisine Linguini with Clam Sauce	1½ LEAN MEAT, 2 STARCH, ½ FAT, ½ VEGETABLE
Romaine lettuce & mushroom salad	½ VEGETABLE

1 tsp olive oil vinegar or lemon juice to taste	1 FAT

Snack

1 cup raw carrot and zucchini slices as desired	1 VEGETABLE
1 cup non-fat fruit yogurt	1 SKIM MILK, 1 FRUIT

Dinner

1 medium artichoke	2 VEGETABLE
1½ oz fresh white fish	1½ LEAN MEAT
½ cup steamed mushrooms	1 VEGETABLE
1/3 cup rice	1 STARCH
½ tsp margarine	½ FAT

Snack

1 cup skim milk	1 SKIM MILK

Exchange Totals for 1,350 kcal/day Diet: #3

	STARCH	LEAN MEAT	VEG	FRUIT	SKIM MILK	FAT	Total
EXCH	5	3.5	5	3	2.5	4	
Carb (g)	82.5	0	25	45	30	0	182.5 g
Pro (g)	16.5	24.5	10	0	20	0	71.0 g
Fat (g)	0	10.5	0	0	tr	20	30.5 g
Kcal	440	192.5	125	180	225	180	1,342.5 kcal

Menu for 1,500 kcal/day Diet: #4

Breakfast
1 slice whole wheat toast — 1 STARCH
1 Tbsp peanut butter — 1 FAT, ½ LEAN MEAT
½ cup skim milk — ½ SKIM MILK
½ medium grapefruit — 1 FRUIT

Snack
1 medium bran muffin — 1 STARCH, 1 FAT
½ cup skim milk — ½ SKIM MILK

Lunch
1½ oz lean roast beef — 1½ LEAN MEAT
2 slices whole wheat bread — 2 STARCH
1½ tsp "light" mayonnaise — ½ FAT
Lettuce, tomato
1 cup steamed broccoli — 2 VEGETABLE
½ cup pineapple juice — 1 FRUIT

Snack
1½ Tbsp wheat germ mixed with — 1 STARCH
8 oz nonfat fruit yogurt — 1 SKIM MILK, 1 FRUIT

Dinner
Spinach, mushroom, bean sprout salad — 1 VEGETABLE
1 tsp oil, plus vinegar to taste — 1 FAT
3½ oz broiled turkey breast — 2 LEAN MEAT
1 cup cooked spaghetti squash — 2 VEGETABLE
½ tsp margarine — ½ FAT
1 baked small potato — 1 STARCH
1 Frozfruit bar — 1 FRUIT

Snack
1 cup skim milk — 1 SKIM MILK

Exchange Totals for 1,500 kcal/day Diet: #4

	STARCH	LEAN MEAT	VEG	FRUIT	SKIM MILK	FAT	Total
EXCH	6	4	5	4	3	4	
Carb (g)	90	0	25	60	36	0	211.0 g
Pro (g)	18	28	10	0	24	0	80.0 g
Fat (g)	0	12	0	0	tr	20	32.0 g
Kcal	480	220	125	240	270	180	1,515.0 kcal

Menu for 1,650 kcal/day Diet: #5

Breakfast

¾ cup bran flakes	1½ STARCH
1 cup skim milk	1 SKIM MILK
½ cup orange juice	1 FRUIT

Snack

½ English muffin	1 STARCH
¼ cup 1% cottage cheese	1 LEAN MEAT
½ cup vegetable juice cocktail	1 VEGETABLE

Lunch

8 (2 oz) boiled medium shrimp	1 LEAN MEAT
½ cup cooked pasta	1 STARCH
2 tsp olive oil, lemon juice to taste	2 FAT
1 cup vegetables such as cucumber, tomato, broccoli, green pepper, etc.	1 VEGETABLE
Mix shrimp, oil, pasta, vegetables.	
1/3 cantaloupe	1 FRUIT

Snack

3 Tbsp wheat germ mixed with 1 cup nonfat fruit yogurt	1 STARCH, 1 SKIM MILK, 1 FRUIT
½ oz (1 slice) 95% fat-free ham	½ LEAN MEAT

Dinner

Romaine lettuce with ½ cup vegetables	½ VEGETABLE
½ tsp oil; vinegar to taste	½ FAT
Tyson Gourmet Selections Chicken Marsala	2 LEAN MEAT, 1½ STARCH, 2 FAT, ½ VEGETABLE
1 cup steamed green beans	2 VEGETABLE
1 medium peach	1 FRUIT
½ cup skim milk	½ SKIM MILK

Snack

3 graham crackers	1 STARCH
½ cup skim milk	½ SKIM MILK

Exchange Totals for 1,650 kcal/day Diet: #5

	STARCH	LEAN MEAT	VEG	FRUIT	SKIM MILK	FAT	Total
EXCH	7	4.5	5	4	3	4.5	
Carb (g)	105	0	25	60	36	0	226.0 g
Pro (g)	21	31.5	10	0	24	0	86.5 g
Fat (g)	0	13.5	0	0	tr	22.5	36.0 g
Kcal	560	247.5	125	240	270	202.5	1,645.0 kcal

Menu for 1,800 kcal/day Diet: #6

Breakfast

1/3 cup *All Bran*	1 STARCH
1 cup skim milk	1 SKIM MILK
½ sliced banana	1 FRUIT
½ whole English muffin	1 STARCH
½ tsp margarine	½ FAT

½ cup tomato juice	1 VEGETABLE

Snack

1 medium corn muffin	1 STARCH, 1 FAT
¼ cup 2% cottage cheese	1 LEAN MEAT
½ cup orange juice	1 FRUIT

Lunch

Celentano Lasagna Primavera	2 LEAN MEAT, 2 STARCH, ½ FAT, 1 VEGETABLE
Romaine salad with 1 cup vegetables	1 VEGETABLE
1 Tbsp reduced calorie salad dressing	½ FAT
1 small orange	1 FRUIT

Snack

1 Tbsp sunflower seeds	1 FAT
1 cup nonfat vanilla yogurt	1 SKIM MILK
6 rye wafers	1½ STARCH

Dinner

2 oz pork loin in oriental stir-fry	2 LEAN MEAT
with 1 cup vegetables of choice	2 VEGETABLE
⅓ cup brown rice	1 STARCH
½ cup *Häagen Dazs* Sorbet & Cream	2 FRUIT, 1½ FAT, ½ SKIM MILK

Snack

½ cup skim milk	½ SKIM MILK

Exchange Totals for 1,800 kcal/day Diet: #6

	STARCH	LEAN MEAT	VEG	FRUIT	SKIM MILK	FAT	Total
EXCH	7.5	5	5	5	3	5	
Carb (g)	112.5	0	25	75	36	0	248.5 g
Pro (g)	22.5	35	10	0	24	0	91.5 g
Fat (g)	0	15	0	0	tr	25	40.0 g
Kcal	600	275	125	300	270	225	1,795.0 kcal

Menu for 2,000 kcal/day Diet: #7

Breakfast

French toast made with 2 slices whole wheat bread,	2 STARCH
¼ cup egg substitute, 1 Tbsp skim milk	1 LEAN MEAT
½ tsp cooking oil	½ FAT
2 Tbsp fruit preserves	½ FRUIT
1 cup skim milk	1 SKIM MILK

Snack

1 slice whole grain bread	1 STARCH
1 Tbsp peanut butter	1 FAT, 1 LEAN MEAT
1 cup nonfat fruit yogurt	1 SKIM MILK, 1 FRUIT

Lunch

Campbell's Chunky Soup Old Fashioned Chicken	1½ MEAT, 1 STARCH, 1 VEGETABLE

6 low-salt crackers	1 STARCH	Large spinach	2 VEGETABLE
½ cup steamed cauliflower	1 VEGETABLE	salad, added vegetables	
15 grapes	1 FRUIT	2 tsp Italian style dressing	1 FAT
Snack		1 slice French bread	1 STARCH
½ bagel	1 STARCH		
1 oz low-fat ricotta cheese	1 LEAN MEAT	1 tsp margarine and garlic	1 FAT
½ cup tomato juice		**Snack**	
½ medium grapefruit	1 FRUIT	1 cup *Yoplait* frozen yogurt	1½ FRUIT, 2 FAT, 1 SKIM MILK
Dinner			
1 cup pasta	2 STARCH		
1 oz lean ground beef	1 LEAN MEAT		
in ½ cup tomato sauce	1 VEGETABLE		

Exchange Totals for 2,000 kcal/day Diet: #7

	STARCH	LEAN MEAT	VEG	FRUIT	SKIM MILK	FAT	Total
EXCH	9	5.5	6	5	3	5.5	
Carb (g)	135	0	30	75	36	0	276.0 g
Pro (g)	27	38.5	12	0	24	0	101.5 g
Fat (g)	0	16.5	0	0	tr	27.5	44.0 g
Kcal	720	302.5	150	300	270	247.5	1,990.0 g

For diets over 2,000 kcal/day, use the exchange plans listed in Chapter 7 for 2,500 and 3,000 kcal/day. The meal plans listed above can be added to or subtracted from, and incorporated into higher or lower calorie diets.

Appendix E Metric Conversions

Weight	To Change	to	Multiply by
	Ounces	Grams	28
	Pounds	Kilograms	0.45
	Grams	Ounces	0.035
	Kilograms	Pounds	2.2

Volume	To Change	to	Multiply by
	Teaspoons	Milliliters	5
	Tablespoons	Milliliters	15
	Fluid ounces	Millilitiers	30
	Cups	Liters	0.24
	Pints	Liters	0.47
	Quarts	Liters	0.95
	Gallons	Liters	3.8
	Milliliters	Fluid ounces	0.03
	Liters	Pints	2.1
	Liters	Quarts	1.06
	Liters	Gallons	0.26

Length	To Change	to	Multiply by
	Inches	Centimeters	2.54
	Feet	Centimeters	30.5
	Yards	Meters	0.9
	Millimeters	Inches	0.04
	Centimeters	Inches	0.4
	Meters	Feet	3.3
	Meters	Yards	1.1

Sample Charts and
Data Collection Forms

Exchange Food Diary   DATE: _____

STARCH	LEAN MEAT	VEG	FRUIT	SKIM MILK	FAT	FOOD TYPES	AMOUNTS
BREAKFAST							
○	○	○	○	○	○		
○	○	○	○	○	○		
○	○	○	○	○	○		
○	○	○	○	○	○		
SNACK							
○	○	○	○	○	○		
○	○	○	○	○	○		
○	○	○	○	○	○		
○	○	○	○	○	○		
LUNCH							
○	○	○	○	○	○		
○	○	○	○	○	○		
○	○	○	○	○	○		
○	○	○	○	○	○		
SNACK							
○	○	○	○	○	○		
○	○	○	○	○	○		
○	○	○	○	○	○		
○	○	○	○	○	○		
DINNER							
○	○	○	○	○	○		
○	○	○	○	○	○		
○	○	○	○	○	○		
○	○	○	○	○	○		
SNACK							
○	○	○	○	○	○		
○	○	○	○	○	○		
○	○	○	○	○	○		
○	○	○	○	○	○		
TOTALS							
___	___	___	___	___	___		

EXAMPLE

Exchange Food Diary 1,200 kcal   DATE: _____

STARCH	LEAN MEAT	VEG	FRUIT	SKIM MILK	FAT	FOOD TYPES	AMOUNTS
BREAKFAST							
●	○	○	○	○	○	Oats	¼ cup
○	○	○	○	●	○	Non-fat yogurt	1 cup
○	○	○	●	○	○	Prunes	3
○	○	○	○	○	◐	Walnuts	1 chopped
SNACK							
○	○	●	○	○	○	Tomato juice	1 cup
○	◐	●	○	○	◐	Jack cheese	½ oz
◐	○	○	○	○	○	Low-salt	3
○	○	○	○	○	○	crackers	
LUNCH							
○	◐	○	○	○	○	95% Fat-free ham	½ oz
○	○	○	○	○	◐	Light mayonnaise	½ Tbsp
●	○	○	○	○	○	Whole wheat bread	1 slice
○	○	●	○	○	○	Raw broccoli/ zucchini	1 cup
SNACK							
○	○	○	●	●	○	Skim milk	1 cup
○	○	○	○	○	○	Banana	½
○	○	○	○	○	○		
○	○	○	○	○	○		
DINNER							
●	●	●	○	○	○	Budget Gourmet Slim Select Glazed Turkey	
●	●	●	○	○	○	Spinach salad	1½ cups
○	○	○	○	○	●	Olive oil	1 tsp
○	○	○	○	○	○	Lemon juice	
SNACK							
○	○	○	◐	◐	●	Breyer's Light	½ cup
○	○	○	◐	○	○	Vanilla ice	
○	○	○	○	○	○	cream	
○	○	○	○	○	○	Blueberries	⅓ cup
TOTALS							
4.5	3	5	3	2.5	3.5		

DATA COLLECTION FORM
SKINFOLD-GIRTH PERCENT BODY FAT ANALYSIS

FEMALES: Sinning Equation-Density/Siri Equation-Percent fat

Name _____   Date _____   Time _____

Age _____   Last Menstrual Period _____

Height (in.) _____   (cm)[in. × 2.54] _____

Weight (lb.) _____   (kg)[lb. × 0.45] _____   GOAL: _____   lb

MEASUREMENTS: (3 at each site; best value is average of closest values)

A. Neck circumference (cm) _____   _____   _____   _____

B. Supra-iliac skinfold (mm) _____   _____   _____   _____

C. Abdominal skinfold (mm) _____   _____   _____   _____

EQUATIONS:

Density = 1.02462 + (0.002024 × A) − (0.001435 × B) − (0.001039 × C)

    1.02462   1.02462

+ (0.002024 × ____cm)   =   + _____

− (0.001435 × ____mm)   =   − _____

− (0.001039 × ____mm)   =   − _____

Total _____   − _____

Percent Fat = [(4.95/Density) − 4.50] × 100

    4.95/ _____   =   _____

− 4.50   =   _____

× 100   =   _____   PERCENT FAT

FAT WEIGHT = Total Weight × [Percent Fat/100]

                 _____ lb × [_____/100] = _____ FAT WEIGHT

LEAN BODY WEIGHT = Total Weight − Fat Weight

                 _____ lb − _____ lb = _____ LEAN BODY WT

DATA COLLECTION FORM
SKINFOLD PERCENT BODY FAT ANALYSIS

MALES: Boscardin Equation-Percent fat

Name _____   Date _____   Time _____

Age _____

Height (in.) _____   (cm)[in. × 2.54] _____

Weight (lb.) _____   (kg)[lb. × 0.45] _____   GOAL: _____   lb

MEASUREMENTS: (3 at each site; best value is average of closest values)

T. Triceps skinfold (mm)   _____   _____   _____   _____

A. Abdominal skinfold (mm) _____   _____   _____   _____

P. Pectoral skinfold (mm)   _____   _____   _____   _____

EQUATIONS:

Percent Fat = 6.036 + (0.446 × T) + (0.279 × A) − (0.486 × P)

$\qquad$ 6.036 $\qquad\qquad$ = $\qquad$ + 6.036

$\qquad$ + (0.446 × _____mm) $\quad$ = $\quad$ + _____

$\qquad$ + (0.279 × _____mm) $\quad$ = $\quad$ + _____

$\qquad$ − (0.486 × _____mm) $\quad$ = $\quad$ − _____

$\qquad$ Total _____ $\qquad$ − _____   PERCENT FAT

FAT WEIGHT = Total Weight × [Percent Fat/100]

$\qquad\qquad$ _____   lb × [_____/100] = _____   FAT WEIGHT

LEAN BODY WEIGHT = Total Weight − Fat Weight

$\qquad\qquad$ _____   lb − _____   lb = _____   LEAN BODY WT

DATA COLLECTION FORM
GIRTH MEASUREMENTS

Name _____ Age _____

INITIAL TEST:

Date _____ Time of Day _____ Last Menstrual Period _____

Height (in.) _____ (cm)[in. × 2.54] _____

Weight (lb.) _____ (kg)[lb. × 0.45] _____ GOAL: _____ lb

MEASUREMENTS: (3 at each site; best value is average of closest values)

1. Upper arm (cm) _____ _____ _____

2. Bust/Chest (cm) _____ _____ _____

3. Waist (cm) _____ _____ _____

4. Hips (cm) _____ _____ _____

5. Mid-thigh (cm) _____ _____ _____

Total _____

FOLLOWUP TEST:

Date _____ Time of Day _____ Last Menstrual Period _____

Height (in.) _____ (cm)[in. × 2.54] _____

Weight (lb.) _____ (kg)[lb. × 0.45] _____ GOAL: _____ lb

MEASUREMENTS: (3 at each site; best value is average of closest values)

1. Upper arm (cm) _____ _____ _____

2. Bust/Chest (cm) _____ _____ _____

3. Waist (cm) _____ _____ _____

4. Hips (cm) _____ _____ _____

5. Mid-thigh (cm) _____ _____ _____

Total _____

References

General References

American Diabetes Association/American Dietetic Association (1986): *Exchange lists for meal planning*. Alexandria, VA: American Diabetes Association, Inc., Chicago: American Dietetic Association.

Bailey, C. (1977). *Fit or fat*. Pleasant Hill, CA: Covert Bailey Publishing Co.

Bennett, W., & Gurin, J. (1982) *The dieter's dilemma*. New York: Basic Books.

Brody, J. E. (1983). *Jane Brody's The New York Times guide to personal health*. New York: Avon Books.

Brody, J. E. (1981). *Jane Brody's nutrition book*. New York: Avon Books.

Brooks, G. A., & Fahey, T. D. (1984). *Exercise physiology: Human bioenergetics and its applications*. New York: John Wiley & Sons.

Committee on Dietary Allowances, Food and Nutrition Board (1980). *Recommended dietary allowances* (9th ed.). Washington, DC: National Academy of Sciences.

Consumer Guide, Editors of (1981). *The dieter's complete guide to calories, carbohydrates, sodium, fats and cholesterol*. New York: Fawcett Columbine.

Fox, E. L., & Mathews, D. K. (1981). *The physiological basis of physical education and athletics* (3rd ed.), Philadelphia: Saunders College Publishing.

Katch, F. I., & McArdle, W. D. (1983). *Nutrition, weight control, and exercise* (2nd ed.). Philadelphia: Lea & Febiger.

Keys, A., Brozek, J., & Henschel, A. (1950). *The biology of human starvation*. Minneapolis: University of Minnesota Press.

Krause, M. V., & Mahan, K. L. (1984). *Food, nutrition, and diet therapy* (7th ed.). Philadelphia: W. B. Saunders.

Remington, D., Fisher, G., & Parent, E. (1983). *How to lower your fat thermostat*. Provo, UT: Vitality House Press, Inc.

Shangold, M. M., & Mirkin, G. (Eds.). (1988). *Women and exercise: Physiology and sports medicine*. Philadelphia: F. A. Davis Company.

Stern, B., Chilnick, L. D., & Sonberg, L. (1987). *The food book*. New York: Dell.

Stryer, L. (1988). *Biochemistry* (3rd ed.). New York: W. H. Freeman.

Stuart, R. B., & Davis, B. (1972). *Slim chance in a fat world.* Champagne, IL: Research Press.

Bibliography

Anderson, D. (1985, May). Eating disorders. *Update: Dance USA,* pp. 9–11. (Available from Dance/USA, 633 E Street NW, Washington, DC 20004.)

Barrow, G. W., & Saha, S. (1988). Menstrual irregularity and stress fractures in collegiate female distance runners. *The American Journal of Sports Medicine, 16,* 209–216.

Belcastro, A. N., & Bonene, A. (1975). Lactic acid removal rates during controlled and uncontrolled recovery exercise. *Journal of Applied Physiology, 36,* 932–936.

Bennett, A. E., Doll, R., & Howell, R. W. (1970). Sugar consumption and cigarette smoking. *Lancet, 1*(7655), 1011–1014.

Benson, J. E., Geiger, C. J., Eisenman, P. A., Wardlaw, G. M. (1989). Relationship between nutrient intake, body mass index, menstrual function, and ballet injury. *Journal of the American Dietetic Association, 1,* 58–63.

Benson, J. E., Gillien, D. M., Bourdet, K., & Loosli, A. R. (1985). Inadequate nutrition and chronic calorie restriction in adolescent ballerinas. *The Physician and Sportsmedicine, 13*(10), 79–90.

Bonato, D. P., & Boland, F. J. (1987): Predictors of weight loss at the end of treatment and one-year follow-up for a behavioral weight loss program. *International Journal of Eating Disorders, 6,* 573–577.

Boscardin, J. B., Schneider, H., Shapiro, R., & Kearney, J. T. (1988). Human body composition measurement: A skin-fold method. *SportCare and Fitness, Nov/Dec,* 11–13.

Bright-See, E., Croy, J., Brayshaw, J., Pearce, D. A., Secker, D. J., & Yoneyama, L. (1978). Nutrition beliefs and practices of ballet students. *Journal of the Canadian Dietetic Association, 39*(4), 324–331.

Brooks-Gunn, J., Warren, M. P., & Hamilton, L. H. (1987). The relation of eating problems and amenorrhea in ballet dancers. *Medicine and Science in Sports and Exercise, 19*(1), 41–44.

Brooks-Gunn, J., & Warren, M. P. (1985). The effects of delayed menarch in different contexts: Dance and nondance students. *Journal of Youth and Adolescence, 14*(4), 285–300.

Brownell, K. D., & Steen, S. N. (1987). Modern methods for weight control. *The Physician and Sportsmedicine, 15*(12), 122–137.

Buono, M. J., Clancey, T. R., & Cook, J. R. (1984). Blood lactate and ammonium ion accumulation during graded exercise in humans. *Journal of Applied Physiology, 57,* 135–139.

Calabrese, L. H., Kirkendall, D. T., Floyd, M., Rapoport, S., Williams, G. W., Weiker, G. G., & Bergfeld, J. A. (1983). Menstrual abnormalities, nutritional patterns, and body composition in female classical dancers. *The Physician and Sportsmedicine. 11*(2), 86–98.

Calabrese, L. H. & Kirkendall, D. T. (1983). Nutritional and medical considerations in dancers. *Clinics in Sports Medicine, 2,* 539–548.

Cann, C. E., Martin, M. C., Genant, H. K., & Jaffe, R. B. (1984). Decreased spinal mineral content in amenorrheic women. *Journal of the American Medical Association, 251,* 626–629.

Chmelar, R. D., Fitt, S. S., Shultz, B. B., Ruhling, R. O., & Shepherd, T. (1988a). Body composition and the comparison of measurement techniques in different levels and styles of dancers. *Dance Research Journal, Summer,* 37–42.

Chmelar, R. D., Shultz, B. B., Ruhling, R. O., Shepherd, T. A., Zupan, M. F., & Fitt, S. S. (1988b). A physiologic profile comparing levels and styles of female dancers. *The Physician and Sportsmedicine, 16*(7), 87–96.

Chmelar, R. D., Fitt, S. S., Shultz, B. B., Ruhling, R. O., & Zupan, M. F. (1987). A survey of health, training, and injuries in different levels and styles of dancers. *Medical Problems of Performing Artists, June,* 61–66.

Clarkson, P. M., Freedson, P. S., Keller, B., Carney, D., & Skrinar, M. (1985). Maximal oxygen uptake, nutritional patterns and body composition of adolescent female ballet dancers. *Research Quarterly for Exercise and Sport, 56,* 180–184.

Cohen, J. L., Kim, C. S., May, P. B. Jr., & Ertel, N. H. (1982a). Exercise, body weight, and professional ballet dancers. *The Physician and Sportsmedicine, 10*(4), 92–101.

Cohen, J. L., Potosnak, L., Frank, O., & Baker, H. (1985). A nutritional and hematologic assessment of elite ballet dancers. *The Physician and Sportsmedicine, 13*(5), 43–54.

Cohen, J. L., Segal, K. R., & McArdle, W. D. (1982b). Heart rate response to ballet stage performance. *The Physician and Sportsmedicine, 10*(11), 120–133.

Cohen, J. L., Segal, K. R., Witriol, I., & McArdle, W. D. (1982c). Cardiorespiratory responses to ballet exercise and the $\dot{V}O_{2\,max}$ of elite ballet dancers. *Medicine and Science in Sports and Exercise, 14,* 212–217.

Dolgener, F. A., Spasoff, T. C., & St. John, W. E. (1980). Body build and body composition of high ability female dancers. *Research Quarterly for Exercise and Sport, 51,* 599–607.

Druss, R. G., & Silverman, J. A. (1979). Body image and perfectionism of ballerinas: Comparison and contrast with anorexia nervosa *General Hospital Psychiatry, 7,* 115–129.

Eisenman, P. A., Johnson, S. C., & Benson, J. E. (1989). *Coaches guide to nutrition and weight control* (2nd ed.). Champagne, IL: Human Kinetics Publishers, Inc.

Epling, W. F., & Pierce, W. D. (1988). Activity-based anorexia: A biobehavioral perspective. *International Journal of Eating Disorders, 7*(4), 475–485.

Fleck, S. J. (1983). Body composition of elite American athletes. *The American Journal of Sports Medicine, 11,* 398–403.

Frisch, R. E., Wyshak, G., Vincent, L. (1980). Delayed menarch and amenorrhea in ballet dancers. *The New England Journal of Medicine, 303*(1), 17–18.

Gladden, L. B. (1989): Lactate uptake by skeletal muscle. *Exercise and Sport Sciences Reviews, 17,* 115–155.

Gleim, G. W., Small, C., Liederbach, M. J., Marino, M., DePasquale, E., & Nicholas, J. A, (1984). Anaerobic power of professional ballet dancers [Abstract]. *Medicine and Science in Sports and Exercise, 16,* 193–194.

Gordon, S. (1981). *Off-balance: The real world of ballet.* New York: McGraw Hill.

Gwinup, G. (1987). Weight loss without dietary restriction: Efficacy of different forms of aerobic exercise. *The American Journal of Sports Medicine, 15,* 275–279.

Hamilton, L. H., Brooks-Gunn, J., Warren, M. P., & Hamilton, W. G. (1988). The role of selectivity in the pathogenesis of eating problems in ballet dancers. *Medicine and Science in Sports and Exercise, 20,* 560–565.

Hamilton, L. H., Brooks-Gunn, J., Warren, M. P., & Hamilton, W. G. (1987). The impact of thinness and dieting on the professional ballet dancer. *Medical Problems of Performing Artists, December,* 117–122.

Hamilton, L. H., Brooks-Gunn, J., & Warren, M. P. (1986). Nutritional intake of female dancers: a reflection of eating problems. *International Journal of Eating Disorders, 5,* 925–934.

Hamilton, L. H., Brooks-Gunn, J., & Warren, M. P. (1985). Sociocultural influences on eating disorders in professional female ballet dancers. *International Journal of Eating Disorders, 4*(4), 465–477.

Harrison, G. G., & Van Italli, T. B. (1982). Estimation of body composition: A new approach based on electromagnetic principles. *American Journal of Clinical Nutrition, 35,* 1176–1179.

Haviland, W. R. (1978). *A physiologic profile of modern dancers.* Unpublished master's thesis, Ohio University, Athens.

Huon, G. F., Brown, L., & Morris, S. (1988). Lay beliefs about disordered eating. *International Journal of Eating Disorders, 7*(2), 239–252.

Kaye, W. H., Enright, A. B., & Lesser, S. (1988). Characteristics of eating disorders programs and common problems with third-party providers. *International Journal of Eating Disorders, 7*(4), 573–579.

Kirkendall, D. T., & Calabrese, L. H. (1983). Physiologic aspects of dance. *Clinics in Sports Medicine, 2,* 525–537.

Klesges, R. C., & Klesges, L. M. (1988). Cigarette smoking as a dietary strategy in a university population. *International Journal of Eating Disorders, 7,* 413–419.

Kvasova, A. P. (1974). Evaluation of a balanced diet for students at a ballet school. *Gigiena; Sanitariya, 8,* 27–29. (From *Nutrition Abstracts Review,* 1975, *45,* 885)

Lloyd, T., Triantafyllou, S. J., Baker, E. R., Houts, P. S., Whiteside, J. A., Kalenak, A., & Stumpf, P. G. (1986). Women athletes with menstrual irregularity have increased musculoskeletal injuries. *Medicine and Science in Sports and Exercise, 18*(4), 374–379.

Loucks, A. B., & Horvath, S. M. (1985). Athletic amenorrhea: A review. *Medicine and Science in Sports and Exercise, 17*(1), 56–72.

Maloney, M. J. (1983). Anorexia and bulimia in dancers: Accurate diagnosis and treatment planning. *Clinics in Sports Medicine, 2,* 549–556.

Marcus, M., Cann, C., Madvis, P., Minkoff, J., Goddard, M., Bayer, M., Martin, M., Ganidan, L., Hashell, W., & Genant, H. (1985). Menstrual function and bone mass in elite women runners. *Annals of Internal Medicine, 102,* 158–168.

Micheli, L. J., Gillespie, W. J., & Walaszek, A. (1984). Physiologic profiles of female professional ballerinas. *Clinics in Sports Medicine, 3,* 199–209.

Mitchell, P. B. (1988). The pharmacological management of bulimia nervosa: A critical review. *International Journal of Eating Disorders, 7*(1), 29–41.

Mostardi, R. A., Porterfield, J. A., Greenberg, B., Goldberg, D., & Lea, M. (1983). Musculoskeletal and cardiopulmonary characteristics of the professional ballet dancer. *The Physician and Sportsmedicine, 11*(12), 53–61.

Nash, H. L. (1985). Body fat measurement: Weighing the pros and cons of electrical impedance. *The Physician and Sports-medicine, 13*(11), 124–128.

Newsholme, E. A. (1980). A possible metabolic basis for the control of body weight. *The New England Journal of Medicine, 302,* 400–405.

Nicholas, J. A. (1975). Risk factors, sports medicine, and the orthopedic system: An overview. *Journal of Sports Medicine and Physical Fitness, 3,* 243–259.

Novak, L. P., Magill, L. A., & Schutte, J. E. (1978). Maximal oxygen intake and body composition of female dancers. *European Journal of Applied Physiology and Occupational Physiology, 39,* 277–282.

Otto, R. M., Parker, C. A., Smith, T. K., Wygand, J. W., & Perez, H. R. (1986). The energy cost of low impact and high impact aerobic dance exercise [Abstract]. *Medicine and Science in Sports and Exercise, 18*(Suppl.), S23.

Oyebode, F., Boodhoo, J. A., & Schapira, K. (1988). Anorexia nervosa in males: Clinical features and outcomes. *International Journal of Eating Disorders, 7,* 121–124.

Passey, R. D., Elson, L. A., & Blackmore, M. (1966). Investigation of the sugar content of cigarettes of different countries. *British Empire Cancer Campaign for Research, Annual Report. 44*(part 2), 6–7.

Pavlou, K. N., Steffee, W. P., Lerman, R. H., & Burrows, B. A. (1985). Effects of dieting and exercise on lean body mass, oxygen uptake, and strength. *Medicine and Science in Sports and Exercise, 17,* 466–471.

Peterson, M. S. (1982). Nutritional concerns for the dancer. *The Physician and Sportsmedicine, 10*(3), 137–143.

Puhl, J. L., & Brown, C. H. (1986). *The menstrual cycle and physical activity.* Champaign, IL: Human Kinetics.

Puhl, J., Case S., Fleck, S., & Van Handel, P. (1982). Physical and physiological characteristics of elite volleyball players. *Research Quarterly for Exercise and Sport, 53,* 257–262.

Puretz, C. D. (1982). Modern dance's effect on the body image. *International Journal of Sports Psychology, 13,* 176–185.

Reeves, R. S., Forey, F. P., & Darnell, L. S. (1986). Effect of exercise and dietary intervention on bodyweight of over-weight adults [Abstract]. *Medicine and Science in Sports and Exercise, 18*(Suppl.), S9.

Rimmer, J. H., & Rosentswieg, J. (1981–82). The maximum O_2 consumption of dance majors. *Dance Research Journal, 14*(1 & 2), 29–31.

Ryan, A. J., & Stephens, R. E. (Eds.) (1989). *The healthy dancer: Dance medicine for dancers.* Princeton, NJ: Dance Horizons/ Princeton Book Company, Publishers.

Ryan, A. J., & Stephens, R. E. (1988). *The dancer's complete guide to healthcare and a long career.* Princeton, NJ: Dance Horizons/ Princeton Book Company, Publishers.

Salkovskis, P. M., Jones, R. Q., Kucyj, M. (1987). Water intoxication, fluid intake, and nonspecific symptoms in bulimia nervosa. *International Journal of Eating Disorders, 6*(4), 524–536.

Schantz, P. G., & Åstrand, P. O. (1984). Physiological characteristics of classical ballet. *Medicine and Science in Sports and Exercise, 16,* 472–476.

Sherman, W. M. (1989). Pre-event nutrition. *Sports Science Exchange, 1*(12). (Available from Gatorade Sports Science Institute, P.O. Box 9005, Chicago, IL 60604-9005.)

Sinning, W. E. (1978). Anthropometric estimation of body density, fat, and lean body weight in women gymnasts. *Medicine and Science in Sports, 10,* 243–249.

Schnitt, J. M., Schnitt, D., & Del A'une, W. (1986). Anorexia nervosa or thinness in modern dance students: comparison with ballerinas. *Annals of Sports Medicine, 3*(1), 9–13.

Vaughan, R., & Snell, P. G. (1986). Physiological variables between elite and good female 10,000 meter runners. *Medicine and Science in Sports and Exercise, 18*(suppl.), S91.

Vincent, L. M. (1989). *Competing with the sylph.* Princeton, NJ: Dance Horizons/Princeton Book Company, Publishers.

Warren, M. P., Brooks-Gunn, J., Hamilton, L. H., Warren, L. F., & Hamilton, W. G. (1986). Scoliosis and fractures in young ballet dancers: Relation to delayed menarche and secondary amenorrhea. *The New England Journal of Medicine, 314*(2l), 1348–1353.

White, L. A. (1982). *Nutritional intake, percent body fat, and physical fitness among professional ballerinas.* Unpublished master's thesis, University of Utah, Salt Lake City.

Wilmore, J. H., Buskirk, E. R., DiGirolamo, M., & Lohman, T. G. (1986). Body composition. *The Physician and Sportsmedicine, 14*(3), 144–162.

Young, V. R., & Scrimshaw, N. S. (1971). The physiology of starvation. *Scientific American, 225*(4), 14–21.

Recommended Cookbooks

Ness, J. Subak-Sharpe, G. (1985). *The calcium-requirement cookbook.* New York: M. Evans & Co.

Weight Watchers International, Inc. (1987). *Weight Watcher's quick and easy menu cookbook*. New York: New American Library.

Weight Watchers International, Inc. (1981). *Weight Watchers 365-day menu cookbook*. New York: New American Library.

Index